the
estrogen
alternative

WHAT EVERY WOMAN NEEDS TO KNOW

ABOUT HORMONE REPLACEMENT

THERAPY AND SERMs, THE NEW

ESTROGEN SUBSTITUTES

Steven R. Goldstein, M.D.
and Laurie Ashner

g. p. putnam's sons
new york

*RG.
186.
.G627
1998*

The suggestions in this book are not intended to replace treatment by
your physician. All questions and concerns regarding your health
should be directed to your physician. The mention of
specific products or brands in this book does not constitute an
endorsement by either the authors or the publisher.
The stories in this book are based on the experiences
of actual people, but the names and circumstances have
been altered to ensure confidentiality.

G. P. Putnam's Sons
Publishers Since 1838
a member of
Penguin Putnam Inc.
375 Hudson Street
New York, NY 10014

Library of Congress Cataloging-in-Publication Data

Goldstein, Steven R.
The estrogen alternative : what every woman needs to know about
hormone replacement therapy and SERMs, the new estrogen substitutes /
Steven R. Goldstein, M.D., and Laurie Ashner.
p.   cm.
ISBN 0-399-14453-6
1. Menopause—Hormone therapy. 2. Selective estrogen receptor
modulators.   I. Ashner, Laurie.   II. Title.
RG186.G627   1998   98-38928 CIP
618.1'75'061—dc21

Printed in the United States of America

1   3   5   7   9   10   8   6   4   2

This book is printed on acid-free paper. ♾

BOOK DESIGN BY JENNIFER ANN DADDIO

To the fabulous women at CCDS and
the miracles they achieve every day
—L.A.

Dedicated to my children, Phoebe and Luke,
and to the hope that in their lifetime medicine
will succeed in pushing the boundaries
of healthy living and healthy lives
to heights beyond all
of our greatest expectations.
—S.R.G.

acknowledgments

This book represents the product of more than three years along a new path on my personal growth curve. I am indebted to the research scientists at Eli Lilly and Company who sought out my advice and counsel (ostensibly because of my expertise in gynecologic ultrasound) to become involved in designing studies to prove uterine safety for Raloxifene. In the process, I realized the vast potential of this category of new compounds known as SERMs (Selective Estrogen Receptor Modulators) for extending postmenopausal women's health. For this I thank Wim Scheele, M.D., Will Dere, M.D., John Termine, Ph.D., Doug Muchmore, M.D., and Hunter Heath, M.D. In addition, the myriad of nonphysician support people who were part of the Raloxifene Heavy Weight team provided an opportunity for me to experience the development of Evista. The excitement of being on the brink of something so new and so important was, in fact, as we say in medicine, "palpable." I want to acknowledge the other members of the gynecology advisory board for Eli Lilly including Anna Parsons, M.D., Patrick Nevin, M.D., Malcolm Whitehead, M.D., Susan Johnson, M.D., Elaine Jolly, M.D., and J. Coen Netelenbos, M.D. I want to acknowledge Elizabeth Haffpapp of the Lotte Burke Method,

Dr. Darrel Rigel (a friend and outstanding dermatologist), as well as Craig Jordan, M.D., for all the useful and helpful information and the time they spent being interviewed by Laurie. I want to thank Laurie Ashner, who is bright, funny, an incredibly quick read, and a perfect co-author. I want to thank Mitch Meyerson, Laurie's husband, who always had a unique insight and helpful comment to offer, Jean Naggar and everyone associated with her agency for their professionalism and perseverance, Karen Bollaert for her assistance and mostly my family—my wife, Kathy, and my children, Phoebe and Luke, for giving me the latitude of time as well as peace of mind to sit down and concentrate and finish the task at hand.

contents

introduction   *1*

ONE
the estrogen dilemma   *5*

TWO
the SERMS *solution*   *37*

THREE
are SERMS *for you?*   *61*

FOUR
raloxifene and how to take it   *91*

FIVE
boosting the benefits   *109*

SIX
natural remedies and SERMS: *should you
try the healing herbs?*   *139*

SEVEN

raloxifene, tamoxifen and beyond:
preventing breast cancer through SERMS   *159*

EIGHT

medicine in the new millennium   *175*

suggested reading   *183*

index   *185*

the estrogen alternative

introduction

In January of 1998 a drug named Raloxifene was released in the United States. It is one of a category of drugs so revolutionary that women suddenly have options in terms of maintaining their long-term health that they have never had before. Raloxifene is marketed by Eli Lilly and Company under the trade name Evista, and the category is called SERMs, Selective Estrogen Receptor Modulators.

What's so revolutionary about SERMs?

These drugs have the potential to allow women everywhere in their postmenopausal years to say good riddance to the estrogen dilemma: "Am I damned if I take it and damned if I don't?" When you stop producing the hormone estrogen at the time of menopause, you must face the choice about whether or not to replace through medication what your body no longer provides. There are clearly tissues where you want and need an estrogenlike function—your heart, your bones, your cholesterol, your brain. There are other tissues where you neither need nor want an estrogen function—your breasts and your uterus. Until now, if you chose to take estrogen, all these tissues were affected.

Consider a woman just past her fiftieth birthday whose mother,

1

aunt and maternal grandmother had breast cancer. Her father and his sister died of heart attacks. Her father's two aunts had hip fractures and ended up in nursing homes. This woman is petrified to take estrogen and petrified not to.

However, women with much less dramatic family medical histories are still in conflict. Many of my patients believe they should be taking estrogen, but they're afraid. They're disheartened by the thought of nuisance bleeding and breast tenderness that are side effects of estrogen replacement therapy. But there is nothing that scares them more than the possibility of an increased chance of breast cancer, a factor that is still disputed widely when it comes to research about estrogen replacement. This is the essence of the estrogen dilemma.

SERMs (*Selective Estrogen Receptor Modulators*) *are one solution to the estrogen dilemma.* Raloxifene, marketed by Eli Lilly and Company under the trade name Evista, can give a woman the estrogenlike function she needs at midlife for her bones and her cholesterol, without fears of it causing breast cancer and uterine cancer. And other SERMs will follow.

Perhaps even more important, SERMs *seem actually to decrease the risks of breast and uterine cancer.* They are capable of acting as an estrogen in bone, heart and cholesterol. They are also a potent antiestrogen in the breast and uterus. The ramifications are endless when you consider that statistics show that among women who live long enough, one in nine will endure breast cancer at some point in her lifetime.

The chapters that follow contain what you need to know about SERMs to decide if they are an option for you. You will learn

- How SERMs work in the body.
- Exactly how SERMs differ from the estrogen supplements currently on the market.

- Why the research that was conducted on Raloxifene can assure you of its safety should you choose to take it.
- Why Evista is currently marketed as osteoporosis prevention rather than a treatment for women in menopause.
- Why one doesn't have to wait ten years to see what happens to women who opt to take Evista or other SERMs that follow to see if there will be side effects.
- How to determine if you are a good candidate for SERMs.
- Beyond estrogen, what else you should be doing to enhance your health.
- What medicine has in store for you once we reach the new millennium, and what is on the cutting edge of research that matters to women in midlife.

If the estrogen dilemma is something that has been troubling you, another alternative is now available. As life expectancy increases, protecting and maintaining her health becomes a woman's greatest priority. An option that millions of women have been waiting for is finally here. In the pages that follow, you will hear the story of SERMs and have the information you need to determine whether or not they can benefit you.

ONE

the estrogen dilemma

At best, it's bad timing. You're asked to make one of the most important decisions about your health when you're not feeling at
your best. Worse, these days everyone, from the co-worker down
the hall to the person who does your manicure, has strong opinions
about what you should do.

Should you take estrogen? Your hairstylist tells you about a
client who gained thirty pounds in three months after she started
to take estrogen. Your neighbor tells you HRT saved her sanity, her
marriage and her waistline. Your doctor tells you that no matter
how well you feel, no matter how much you diet, exercise and
take care of yourself, you'll do the best for your body, your bones
and your heart by replacing the estrogen your body no longer
makes.

You decide to read whatever you can get your hands on and
think for yourself. But everything you read seems contradictory.
The medications to treat the symptoms of this time of life have
names that make you grit your teeth or laugh out loud. You remember what you really hated about high-school biology class.

One thing is for sure: When you've reached menopause and are
considering the benefits and drawbacks of taking estrogen, you

aren't alone if you're petrified to take it and petrified not to. In truth, most women are confused about what they should do.

Kris is a case in point. At five A.M., five mornings a week, she pulls on her sweats and T-shirt, grabs the overstuffed tote she filled the night before with her outfit for work, and heads to her health club. It's one of the nation's top facilities, filled with chrome and mirrors, state-of-the-art Cybex equipment and crowds of people. It's a place to see and be seen, but Kris prays she won't see anyone she knows so she can get through her routine quickly. She can't stop and chat. She has to get on the highway early enough or a twenty-minute commute will turn into an hour.

Making time for exercise each morning has taken enormous self-discipline. Her menopause came two years ago. Already she's lost 3 percent of her bone mass. Her cholesterol doesn't look great. But she didn't do well on HRT. "The progesterone made me feel sick," she says. "I felt bloated and irritable, my breasts ached, and I just hated it." She's off it now, but she's worried about whether or not she made the right decision. "My mother died of a heart attack at sixty-four. I worry about that happening to me. The idea that my bones are thinning this fast scares me, too. Still, I can't be sick and miserable all the time. I'm going the so-called natural, or exercise route."

Marla, fifty-one, would agree. She decided to try HRT. She had a prescription for Premarin in her purse when she heard that her younger cousin was diagnosed with breast cancer at forty-three.

"Now I'm completely confused," Marla admits. "When you see this happen to a healthy woman with young children, why would any woman want to take an unnecessary gamble and raise her chances? There are so many things that we do that might eventually cause cancer. Why should I take on one more? So I'm not going to take estrogen for now. When I wake up in a sweat, I have a meditation I do to fall back to sleep and a tea I drink which helps sometimes."

But is she satisfied with her choice? She shrugs, uncomfortably. "My skin is so dry, I'm noticing new lines every day. I don't want to end up looking like eighteen miles of burned-out highway." She stops for a moment and slides her bracelet back and forth, working it over the widest part of her hand. "Sometimes I get hot flashes I can't hide. My face goes bright red. Still, I'm doing everything I can do." She sighs. "Everything but take estrogen."

Rebecca, fifty-four, made a different choice. She's been on hormone replacement therapy since the beginning of her menopause. When tests showed that her body was no longer making estrogen, she was feeling great, otherwise. She'd been exercising and eating a low-fat diet for years and was reaping the results. Still, it was the preventive and health-maintenance aspects of estrogen replacement therapy that drew her to the treatment. "It might sound vain, but I want to look young and stay active as long as I can. Let's face it, my skin, my hair, my sex life—these things matter to me and I know estrogen helps. Still, the thought of taking these pills for the rest of my life doesn't thrill me. I wonder if I'm going to pay for this later."

Lauren was sixty-two years old the first time she felt a strange tightness in her chest. "It was just a tiny bit of pain. I'd played a couple of sets of tennis that morning and I thought I might have pulled a muscle. The pain went away, but when it happened again three days later, I called my doctor.

"Of course, you know how it always goes. By the time you get to the doctor's office, you feel absolutely fine. He made me walk on a treadmill and looked at my blood pressure. He told me that I don't really have heart disease, but since I have a family history of it, I should definitely be on HRT.

"My menopause was really no big deal; I never felt a need for HRT. But, if it was going to be good for my heart, I thought, I might as well. So I tried it. First thing I know, my breasts ache so badly, I can't sleep on my stomach, which means I can't sleep at all. Two weeks later, I'm playing tennis, and all of a sudden, I'm having a period. Try to find a tampon or a Kotex in a retirement community in Florida at two o'clock in the afternoon on a Tuesday. There's no one there under sixty. Finally I remember the young girl who runs the pro shop. She finds a minipad in her locker. I think, "This is HRT? This is nuts."

I have met many women like Lauren, Rebecca, Marla and Kris in the course of my practice. There are 37 million women in the U.S. who are in or past menopause. Twenty million more will reach menopause in the next ten years. All these women will face the decision about whether or not to replace the estrogen their body no longer provides on its own.

The majority of my patients who have reached menopause know on one level or another that there are some benefits from taking estrogen. They're well-read. They've heard that taking estrogen can keep their bones strong and lower their risk of heart disease (factors I will go into in depth later in this chapter). But they're afraid. They're put off by the thought of nuisance bleeding and breast tenderness. But they are truly frightened because of the current dispute about whether HRT increases a woman's chance of breast cancer. Even my patients who opt for HRT are still enormously conflicted.

This is the heart of the estrogen dilemma: In 1850 a woman became menopausal at an average age of forty-six and often died at age fifty. But life expectancy for a woman now fifty years old who doesn't already have cancer or heart disease is ninety-one. As life expectancy continues to increase, your chances of living one-third or more of your life in postmenopause and an estrogen-deprived state are also increasing.

There are as many as three hundred different tissues in a woman's body equipped with estrogen receptors, chemical sites that are responsive to estrogen. That means that estrogen levels in the body affect a broad range of tissues and organs. There are clearly tissues where you want and need an estrogenlike function—your heart, your bones, your cholesterol, your brain. There are other tissues where you don't need nor want an estrogen function—your breasts and your uterus. Unfortunately, the most popular forms of HRT that doctors prescribe deliver estrogen to all those tissues.

For a medical treatment as well-known as HRT, the numbers of women who choose not to follow the regimen or who drop it after the first year or so are astounding. Researchers estimate that only about 20 percent of the 37 million menopausal and post-menopausal women in the USA take HRT. Many of those women use HRT for a year or more, and of those half stop within two years.

I've begun to realize that my patients are making their choices according to what they are most afraid of, a sad way to choose what to do for your health. If they are most afraid of breast cancer, they shy away from HRT. If they fear breaking bones or heart disease, they shy away from doing nothing, and opt for HRT. It's again something at the heart of the dilemma—there's no hundred-percent right decision and no hundred-percent wrong decision. And then there are women who try to do what they know is best for their health, take HRT and do so poorly on it, they can't continue.

Let's take a closer look at the estrogen dilemma.

WHY TAKE ESTROGEN,
EVEN IF I FEEL FINE?

Women come into my office who are clearly menopausal, clearly making no estrogen. They are exercising, eating healthily, and doing all the right things to stay healthy, and they feel great. But I have to tell them that there's no question that however well they're doing, estrogen replacement will improve their cholesterol and be good for their heart and bones. There are two issues to keep in mind when you think about estrogen replacement. One is taking it to relieve symptoms. The other is taking it to maintain long-term health, even though you may have no symptoms.

Until now, estrogen replacement therapy was the best medical science had to offer to achieve both goals. Here's why.

• **Estrogen and your heart:** In survey after survey, women list breast cancer or other cancer as their primary health concern. But heart disease is still the number-one killer of women. One in three women over sixty-five will develop the disease. It is estimated that 500,000 women a year die from coronary artery disease. That is twice as many women as die each year from cancer.

Women seem to have a built-in protection against cardiovascular disease while they are menstruating. How soon do women catch up with men's rate of heart disease once their bodies stop producing estrogen? Researchers say fifteen years. For a woman who reaches menopause at the average age of fifty-one, this means she will be sixty-six—relatively young by today's standards. Keep in mind that heart disease doesn't always mean a fatal heart attack. It can be a debilitating disease that seriously restricts you.

In the recent Nurses' Health Study, which has been following the health of 120,000 nurses for more than a decade, researchers

islands. My husband kept saying, 'It's not that hot. Look at the temperature.' All I could think was that seventy degrees on the Greek islands must mean something different than seventy degrees in Greenwich, Connecticut, because I was burning up. Anyway, that's how I learned about hot flashes."

Hot flashes are one well-known result of the loss of estrogen. Let's take a closer look at the hot flash, for a moment.

Hot flashes fall under the category doctors call "vasomotor instability." When your supply of estrogen dwindles, the hypothalamus, the "temperature regulation control station" in the brain, goes awry. It sends a message to the pituitary gland to send out a hormone to stimulate the ovaries to produce more estrogen. This hormone is known as follicle stimulating hormone (FSH). When the ovaries do not respond because of menopause, the hypothalamus can sometimes release a stimulant called free epinephrine. This spills over into the heat-regulating area and the result is increased circulation, dilated blood vessels—a hot flash. Blood rushes to the skin. You flush. The sensation can quickly travel through your whole body.

These "flashes" or "flushes" may last from thirty seconds to thirty minutes. Some women have only a few episodes a year, but there are women who have them daily, and often. There are women who have suffered with twenty or more such flashes a day.

Hot flashes, while uncomfortable, are not medically dangerous to you. And they are not forever. In about two-thirds of women, hot flashes last from one to five years. About one-quarter of women will experience hot flashes for up to ten years. Fewer than 10 percent will experience them for more than ten years.

Women who have a surgical menopause (surgical removal of the ovaries) often suffer the most from frequent hot flashes. This is probably because the drop in estrogen levels in these women is so abrupt and complete. However, hot flashes and night sweats may lead to insomnia, irritability, fatigue and mood swings.

• **Estrogen and your longevity:** *The New England Journal of Medicine* published a study in June 1997 which reported that women who take hormone replacement therapy for ten years reduce their risk of dying from all causes by 37 percent. The study followed 60,000 postmenopausal women for sixteen years. The percent drops to 20 percent beyond ten years.

• **Estrogen and your bones:** There are 206 bones in your body. They give you support, they allow you to go about your daily activities, and they protect your vital organs. Bone marrow even manufactures new blood cells. Although you many think of bone as inert and unchanging, it is living tissue, and like all living tissue is constantly changing, breaking down old cells, and replacing them with new cells, resorped as well as formed. Your bone mass, which is the total amount of bone in your skeleton, is maintained in a delicate balance between the breakdown (resorption) of old bone and the formulation of new bone.

From the time you are born until you reach early adulthood, you produce much more new bone tissue than you lose through bone breakdown. Around age thirty-five, however, your body reaches skeletal maturity. Medically this is known as peak bone mass. After this point, an imbalance in the bone remodeling system begins so that old bone removal outpaces replacement of new bone.

Ninety-nine percent of the calcium in your body is stored in your bones. Calcium is so vital to the human body that there is an elaborate system of hormones to ensure that there is always enough of it in your blood. Estrogen promotes the body's use of calcitonin and parathyroid hormones, as well as vitamin D. All these biochemical reactions influence bone health. Estrogen also plays a role in keeping the blood calcium levels normal by aiding absorption of calcium from food as well as promoting the uptake of calcium from the blood into the bone.

After menopause, your body may lose bone faster than it can be replaced due to estrogen loss. Fifty percent of a woman's bone loss occurs in the first three years following menopause. Some women lose up to one-third of the bone mass in their spine in as little as six years after menopause. This bone loss defines osteopenia and osteoporosis.

The bone disease of osteoporosis (weak or thin bones), or its precursor of low bone mass known as osteopenia, can lead to spine, wrist, and hip fracture in later years resulting from bones continually losing density and strength. Twenty-five million Americans suffer from osteoporosis.

It's known as the silent disease because there are no symptoms that this is happening at first. If they do nothing to stop the process, about 25 percent of postmenopausal women will develop osteoporosis and be at risk for fractures as they age. A woman is at highest risk for fracture during her eighties.

The National Osteoporosis Foundation has shared these findings:

- One in four women will develop osteoporosis and nearly 50 percent of all women over the age of fifty will sustain an osteoporosis-related fracture.

- More than 1.3 million bone fractures currently occur each year in U.S. women.

- One out of every six women will suffer a hip fracture in her lifetime, a risk equal to the combined risks of developing breast, uterine, and ovarian cancer.

- In terms of hip fractures, the rate for women is two to three times higher than that for men.

- Twenty percent of postmenopausal women who experience hip fractures die within one year of the injury and 50 percent of those who survive never walk independently again.

- Two hundred thousand women will experience a wrist fracture each year.

- As the population ages, the prevalence of osteoporosis will double by the year 2020.

Once you get osteoporosis, you cannot reverse it completely. Thus it is important to prevent it before it happens. Unfortunately, you can consume 1,500 mg of calcium every day and make it a point to do weight-bearing exercise three times a week, but if you don't replace your estrogen, you will still lose bone mass no matter how consistent you are. Mounting evidence suggests that taking estrogen along with progesterone immediately after menopause can go a long way toward preventing bone loss. Estrogen replacement has been shown to significantly decrease fracture risk in postmenopausal women. Estrogen's role is to stop some bone resorption—the process that decreases bone density. Estrogen replacement is the most potent antiresorptive available today and, until recently, the only real choice.

• **Estrogen and your emotions:** Does dwindling estrogen really have anything to do with mood swings? While researchers maintain that there is no direct link between menopause and depression, they have found that estrogen has a mental tonic effect. It enhances moods—especially for women who take estrogen and testosterone together. In fact, estrogen replacement therapy has been found to reduce anxiety, one frequent complaint of women who have reached menopause.

While menopause may not cause depression, many doctors feel that women at this stage are more vulnerable to it because of their fluctuating hormones, especially at the time of transition into menopause, known as perimenopause.

• **Estrogen and sexual interest:** Too busy, too bored, too tired, or too little estrogen? Estrogen stimulates the creation of the vagina's tough, outer layer of cells, known as the epithelium, that protects the delicate tissues underneath. It also moistens the vaginal mucus membranes, which increases lubrication.

A patient I'll call Caroline remarried four years ago at the age of fifty-five. This is what she had to say about estrogen and sex: "I think people play down how dry a woman gets after menopause because sex at this age was a topic women weren't openly discussing until now. I thought dry would mean what it used to mean when you weren't turned on with a man and you had to work a little harder at it. No one told me how dry you actually get and how difficult sex really becomes. For me, it just keeps getting worse. Astroglide helped, but my older sister told me, "Wait. In another year, even that isn't going to do you much good." Worse, I'm getting one bladder infection after another. My doctor told me that without estrogen replacement, the tissues will continue to get dry and can be easily injured during sex. The whole topic makes me mad. I'm no feminist, but if men were losing testosterone this fast and they couldn't have sex, they'd be selling totally safe doses of synthetic testosterone where you get your Sunday paper."

If you don't replace estrogen, blood flow to the vagina decreases and it will eventually take longer to become sexually aroused or to become lubricated enough to have comfortable sex. As time goes on, the vagina becomes thinner, narrower, less elastic.

Yes, having frequent sex may help you stay more interested and able, and help maintain muscle tone in the vagina. True, lubricants such as Replens or Astroglide can be godsends. But eventually, without estrogen, the changes that make sex uncomfortable happen to every woman.

Women who do not replace estrogen after menopause often encounter a change in the pH level in the vagina, making it more alkaline. This is more favorable for some infections. The support system of these internal organs can weaken, causing prolapse of the uterus. All of this, obviously, can interfere with your sex life.

• **Estrogen and your skin:** Estrogen receptors have been identified on the skin cells that manufacture collagen, the main protein in the skin that is thought to keep skin plump. A loss of collagen results in wrinkling and thinning of the skin and a greater tendency to bruise. While it won't turn back the clock, estrogen helps preserve collagen, which keeps skin moist.

• **Estrogen and your hair:** There's no amount of gels and shampoos that will tame it and there's so much of it in your brush that you fear you're losing your hair. What's happening here? Estrogen maintains the growth and rest cycle of the health of each hair. Hair loss can be due to stress—but it can also be due to your body's adaptation to the loss of estrogen.

• **Estrogen and your sleep:** Women who take estrogen fall asleep faster, sleep longer and have fewer episodes of wakefulness during the night.

• **Estrogen and your teeth:** Women taking hormone replacement therapy suffer a lower incidence of tooth loss, due to better skeletal bone health.

IF ESTROGEN DOES ALL THESE MARVELOUS THINGS, WHY DO SO MANY WOMEN REFUSE TO TAKE IT?

One patient told me: "I have this picture that HRT means swallowing a huge estrogen tablet each day and having it go racing through my bloodstream causing some kind of hormonal buzz."

It doesn't work that way. The amount of estrogen prescribed is not a full replacement. The dose of estrogen most doctors prescribe is about 0.625 mg per day. That's a fraction of the amount of estrogen that your ovary used to produce. It's one-half of the amount of effective estrogen contained in the ultra–low dose birth control pills such as Loestrin 1/20 or Alesse and nowhere near the amount of estrogen you added to your body if you took the birth control pills available when you were in your twenties. If your mother took estrogen when she reached menopause, she took four to ten times as much as what doctors prescribe for women today. Still, today's small dosage is usually enough to relieve you of the two major symptoms of lack of estrogen women come to see their gynecologists about: vaginal dryness and hot flashes.

When I prescribe HRT, it's after a long discussion, where I help a woman weigh her risks and benefits. Then I design a treatment specifically for her. The prescription for HRT often requires a little fine-tuning. Women differ in their sensitivity to estrogen, and doses need to be adjusted according to a woman's weight or age, for example. Some women simply require a higher dose to relieve their symptoms, especially those who have menopause at an age younger than the average of fifty-one, or if the menopause is surgically induced by a hysterectomy. The best hormone therapy gives a woman the minimum amount of medication she needs for maximum benefits.

Today estrogen is prescribed in three ways: tablets, patches and vaginal inserts.

Tablets. Premarin, made by Wyeth Ayerst, is the most widely prescribed estrogen in pill form in the United States today. When you hear of a study on women taking estrogen, it is usually Premarin that was being researched, since it has been on the market since 1941.

Premarin is manufactured from the urine of pregnant horses. The usual dose is 0.625 mg, although 0.9 mg is also commonly used for women whose menopausal symptoms, such as frequent hot flashes, night sweats or dry vagina, don't respond to the lower dose.

Estrace and Ogen are two other commonly prescribed estrogen tablets. Estrace comes from a natural plant compound and contains either 0.5 or 1.0 mg of ethinyl estradiol. Ogen comes from modified plant estrogen and contains 0.625 mg of estrogen.

Skin patches. These small, round, self-adhesive skin patches deliver estradiol through the skin directly into the bloodstream continuously and gradually. The most common skin patches prescribed are Estraderm, Climara and Vivelle. They come from natural plant compounds.

Because estrogen is not being taken orally when women use "the patch," the drug bypasses the liver. However, most of the positive effect on cholesterol that women taking Premarin experience occurs initially in the liver. So women on the patch will not get this full benefit.

These patches are worn on the buttocks or abdomen continuously, even while bathing or swimming. They need to be changed once or twice a week, depending on the brand.

Vaginal inserts:

Creams. Premarin is also available as a cream that a woman can insert directly into her vagina. Ogen, Estrace and Dienstrol are other frequently prescribed creams. Creams relieve vaginal dryness, but they have a relatively low absorption rate into the circulatory system. Creams aren't usually enough to prevent bone loss or heart disease or to provide the other protections of estrogen in tablet form.

The Ring. Estring is a new option for women dealing with the aggravating problem of vaginal dryness. It's a ring, placed in the vagina, that releases estradiol. It's easy and it's comfortable. It isn't absorbed systemically, which means you won't find higher levels of estrogen in your blood. My patients love it, and when I have tested their blood for increased levels of estrogen, the result is negative.

Beyond fears about the risk of breast cancer, which I'll go into in a moment, women have other complaints about HRT. These are some of the complaints I hear most often:

• **The progesterone phase can be uncomfortable (and downright intolerable for some).**

When a woman takes estrogen alone (pills, patches and even sometimes creams), the endometrium (lining of the uterus) grows and thickens. This can create a higher risk for developing endometrial hyperplasia (precancer) and cancer. This is why doctors recommend that women taking estrogen also take progestin, which causes the uterine wall to slough off, eliminating the risk. The most widely prescribed progesterone supplement is Provera. You can take one capsule that contains both estrogen and progesterone, or you can take progesterone as a separate pill. Other oral progestins include Aygestin and Cycrin. Prometrium is a new brand that utilizes micronized natural progesterone.

Many women take sequential HRT. This means progesterone is also prescribed with the estrogen unless the patient has had a hysterectomy, in which case the progesterone isn't needed. Think of estrogen as the "good guy." You take it daily. The progestin is then taken either for ten to twelve to fourteen days per month in a dose of 10 mg per day (although recently doctors have been reducing it to 5 mg a day.) Unfortunately a lot of women can't tolerate that dose of progesterone for that period of time because it causes breast tenderness and mood swings. As one patient put it, "My husband has this thing he does when I'm doing the dishes. He sneaks up behind me and puts his arms around me and grabs my breasts. When he did it while I was on progesterone, I almost yelped. 'Get away from me!' I screamed. Since he's been doing this for twenty years and it usually makes me laugh, he looked at me like I'd really lost it." Women also complain of cramps, irritability, and two weeks of PMS while taking progesterone.

• **You continue to get a "period."**

Most women will have a withdrawal bleed on this regimen after day 9, 10, 11 or 12 relative to the ten days of progestin therapy. This means you can be sixty years old and ostensibly still be getting a monthly period.

There is a newer regimen. It involves taking a smaller dose of progestin all the time. Wyeth now markets a drug called Prempro, a combination of Premarin 0.625 mg and either 2.5 mg or 5 mg medroxyprogesterone acetate (or MPA, the generic form of Provera). With Prempro there's no estrogenic buildup, so 60 to 70 percent of women have no further bleeding. The problem is if you do bleed, there is no schedule. Therefore, if you do experience any vaginal bleeding, you need an examination because of the potential that there could be an abnormality. This newer approach seems to work better in older women who are years past the beginning of menopause and who want to avoid periods.

Another approach being tried is a type of cyclical HRT regimen where women take estrogen continuously but progesterone is added only once every three months. Therefore they go two months without a period, then bleed in the third month, which means only four periods a year. The bleeding is usually a couple of days longer and heavier, however, when they do have a withdrawal bleed. This method of HRT is being studied for long-term safety, so it's important to discuss it with your doctor. I use transvaginal ultrasound in these patients to demonstrate that their lining has indeed thinned.

• **Estrogen pills may aggravate existing medical problems.** These conditions include liver and gallbladder disease, migraine headaches, high blood pressure and high blood trigylcerides. If you have a history of endometriosis, a condition where the uterine lining spreads and attaches itself to other organs, estrogen replacement may cause a recurrence.

• **You have to continue to take estrogen for years to get the long-term benefits of protection from osteoporosis and heart disease.** To prevent osteoporosis, for instance, a woman must use estrogen continuously for at least seven years, according to new research. If you've only been taking it to ward off menopausal symptoms such as hot flashes and sleeplessness, when these symptoms end—for many women that's two to three years—you may not want to continue the discomfort for such goals as better bones and reduced risk of heart disease. This is especially true if you aren't in high-risk categories.

Yet the preventive properties of estrogen stop when you stop taking it. Suppose you begin taking HRT at age fifty. If you stop at fifty-five, you can't expect your bones to be protected from osteoporosis when you turn seventy.

• **Some women experience side effects.**

Women sometimes get breast tenderness from fluid retention. There can also be fluid retention elsewhere in the body. Some women complain of dark spots on their chest and neck. Jean, fifty-one, says, "I wanted HRT because I had such hot flashes and so much moodiness that I was willing to try just about anything. I was on Premarin, and when I complained that my breasts felt heavy and swollen, the doctor but me on Prempro. With this form of HRT I'd have no periods, she explained, and maybe my breasts would feel better. Two months later, I'm fifteen pounds heavier. 'You're retaining water,' she told me. 'I'm retaining everything,' I complained. She suggested some vitamins that might help with the water retention. Great. Now I'm running to the bathroom twice an hour. I'm still bloated. I complained again, and she shook her head and sighed and reminded me once again about the benefits of estrogen—good for my bones, good for my cholesterol, good for my menopausal symptoms. I left feeling depressed, thinking, 'I'll have great bones but I'll never be able to zip anything I own again.' "

• **Many women will find that they're simply disenfranchised. They can't take HRT even if they want to.** It is not advised for women with a history of breast or uterine cancer. It is not recommended for women with clotting problems. They cannot and should not take hormone replacement therapy, even if they want to.

WHAT IS THE TRUTH ABOUT
BREAST CANCER AND HRT?

Central to the debate over HRT is whether or not it increases breast cancer. Again, there are tissues where you clearly want estrogen (bone, lipids) and tissues where you definitely don't. The breast tissue is one area where you definitely do not want more estrogen.

The most frequent question I hear from patients when I suggest HRT remains, "Will I get breast cancer?" What are your real chances of getting breast cancer if you take HRT? The general incidence for breast cancer rises for every woman over time. Women between the ages of seventy to seventy-nine have 24 percent of all cases. General risk factors for developing breast cancer include starting menstruation before age twelve, reaching menopause after age fifty-five, and having either no children or your first child after age thirty, genetic predisposition, which means having a mother or sister with the disease, obesity, smoking and environmental factors. Still, breast cancer occurs in women with no known risk factors at all.

Although 46,000 women die annually from breast cancer, the survival rate has never been better. The disease is now highly treatable if detected in its earliest stages. Women with localized breast cancer—i.e., it has not spread to anywhere else in the body— experience a 97 percent five-year survival rate. The five-year survival rate for all stages of breast cancer is now 84 percent.

But what happens when women take estrogen? The central argument is that estrogen "nudges" breast cells to divide, which can heighten cancer risk. Studies, sometimes published only months apart, have contradicted each other about whether there really is a risk, or whether the benefits outweigh the risks.

The Nurses' Health Study has been tracking 121,700 meno-pausal women in the United States for twenty years. The study began in 1976, when these women were thirty to fifty-five years old. *The New England Journal of Medicine* published an interim re-port in June 1997. Based on the study's findings, they estimated that in the first ten years, women on hormone therapy had a 24 percent reduced risk of dying from breast cancer.

However, after ten years, the risk of death from breast cancer was increased by 43 percent over that of women who had not taken hormones. Another finding was that women on HRT who had a family history of breast cancer had no greater risk of devel-oping breast cancer than women with no family history of breast cancer. And women who did get breast cancer while they were in the first ten years of HRT had a lower death rate than women who never took hormones, which researchers attribute to earlier detection among hormone users who seem to see their doctors more often. The final results won't be out until the year 2005. However, critics already point out that this study depends on self-reported data—women merely complete questionnaires every two years.

The Centers for Disease Control and Prevention did their own study and found a 30 percent increase in the risk of breast cancer after fifteen years of estrogen use.

Then several studies were published where researchers pooled all the available research from other smaller studies. These stud-ies didn't provide new data but reinterpreted the data that had al-ready been released from other studies. A study published in *Lancet*, a British medical journal, in 1997 analyzed fifty-one world-wide studies. Their results? Of women who began using HRT at age fifty, two additional cases of breast cancer occurred in a thou-sand women who used HRT for five years. There were six occurrences per thousand in women using HRT for ten years and twelve occurrences per thousand women after fifteen years. That's less than a 1 percent increase.

The *Journal of the American Medical Association* published a study by doctors at the University of Washington in Seattle that showed HRT was not associated with an increased risk for breast cancer.

A study published in the journal *Contraception* is also of great interest. Two hundred researchers brought together virtually all the studies ever done on the subject of the pill and breast cancer. Those studies included data from 153,536 women from twenty-five countries. They found that there was no increased chance of being diagnosed with breast cancer ten to twenty years after stopping the use of the pill.

Granted, the pill and HRT are not the same thing. But the study is reassuring because these are long-term results from a significant population involving pills containing a higher dose of estrogen than those usually prescribed for HRT. But it's a lower dose than their own bodies would have made off the pill.

When evaluating these studies, keep the following in mind:

- No studies have shown any increased risk for breast cancer from short-term (less than five years) use of HRT.

- None of the studies on HRT are prospective, randomized, placebo-controlled studies, the gold standard of scientific research.

- It isn't easy to study breast cancer. It's a disease that takes a long time to develop. A study has to follow women for a very long time and there are lifestyle issues, such as smoking, drinking or weight gain, that are also relevant and affect a woman's chances of developing breast cancer. It's difficult to take all the other factors out and study just one.

My position on HRT and breast cancer is that I believe estrogen, at least in long-term use in postmenopausal women, is a *promoter* of breast cancer, not an *inducer* or cause. Looking at the Nurses' Health Study data, which have perhaps received the most media attention, we see a 30 to 40 percent increase in breast cancer in postmenopausal women after ten years of use. To those of us struggling to get double-digit returns on our retirement funds, this sounds like an astronomical number. Realize, however, that this is a relative risk of 1.3 times the baseline. In scientific studies, when one thing actually *causes* another, you expect to see relative risks of four-, five- or sixfold increases. For example, the relative risk of cigarette smoking and lung cancer is a forty-two-fold increase, or 4,200 percent, or a relative risk of 42.0. Therefore I do not believe that estrogen is the cause of breast cancer, but I do believe that if the cancer is beginning to develop, estrogen will promote it.

Finally there is a well-designed, long-term study under way. In 1995, the National Institutes of Health launched a $628-million Women's Health Initiative. The HRT portion of the study involves 27,500 women. Half of the women are receiving HRT, the other half a placebo. Within the group taking HRT are subgroups taking different *kinds* of HRT, so this study has the potential to generate a wealth of specific information. The researchers will compare these women's rates of heart disease, breast cancer and osteoporosis over at least an eight-year period. This is a study to watch. Trouble is, you'll have to wait until the year 2005 to hear the results.

THE NEW OPTION: SERMS—
SELECTIVE ESTROGEN RECEPTOR
MODULATORS—ESTROGEN ALTERNATIVES
FOR THE TWENTY-FIRST CENTURY

Imagine drugs that act as estrogen for heart, bone and cholesterol, while being potent antiestrogens in the breast and uterus. With such drugs, whatever one's genetic and/or environmental risk factors are, they are actually diminished. Furthermore, if they don't stimulate the lining of the uterus, there is no monthly bleeding and no need for progesterone to protect against endometrial hyperplasias and cancers.

A new drug that appears to act this way actually exists. It is called Raloxifene, made by Eli Lilly and Co. of Indianapolis and marketed as Evista.

There is no doubt in my mind that ultimately these selective estrogen receptor modulators will make many of our current approaches obsolete, but as you will learn, they aren't for everybody, and the more knowledge you have, the more confident your personal decision will be.

The estrogen dilemma doesn't end after the first few years of menopause. In fact, the estrogen dilemma is greater for women the longer they live postmenopause. There is a difference between taking estrogen to relieve nuisance symptoms and taking it for health maintenance. Health maintenance will become an even bigger issue in the year 2000 as life expectancy increases and the quality of life in those extra years is the goal. It is no longer enough to live to be ninety-one. You have to hope now that when you are eighty-five, you'll be as healthy and active as a sixty-five-year-old person is today. Otherwise, why bother? And if you want to be strong and vital and able to do things you want to do and not just "be alive," preservation of your health is the key. That means preventing osteoporosis, preventing heart disease, reducing cholesterol, and, it is hoped, preventing Alzheimer's disease, while reducing risks of breast and uterine cancer.

QUESTIONS WOMEN ASK

How soon can one expect to feel better after starting HRT?

Side effects such as vaginal dryness, hot flashes and night sweats disappear almost immediately, definitely within weeks, for 90 percent of women taking estrogen. Trouble concentrating, forgetfulness and anxiety usually are relieved within a month. HRT sometimes enhances a woman's sex drive, because it makes her feel so much better otherwise. Sleep problems that were caused by low estrogen levels will also clear up, usually within a month. In addition, after several months on HRT you should notice less dryness of your skin and hair.

I was adopted at birth, and I don't know my family history. Is there some test I can take to see if I'm at greater risk for osteoporosis or heart disease, or whether I should take any kind of hormone replacement therapy, including HRT?

In my experience, people who are adopted and do not have a family history often assume the worst in terms of their genetic predispositions so they won't be caught off guard. However, when it comes to hormone replacement therapy, making that assumption creates a great dilemma. For instance, if you have a strong family history of heart disease as well as osteoporosis and breast cancer but you aren't aware of it because of your adoption, what should you do?

Your doctor can help you evaluate your personal history for some clues. Here's what I'd want to know as your physician, at the minimum: What is your age? Are you or were you ever a smoker? Are you slight and thin? Have you ever fractured a bone? Have you had any thyroid disease or prolonged use of corticosteroids for other medical problems? Have you had long episodes of lack of menses in your younger years? What is your cholesterol? How is your blood pressure? Do you exercise regularly? Do you maintain a low-fat diet?

Not knowing one's family history is difficult in the perimenopausal and postmenopausal years, but you will learn in the following chapters that given your own special estrogen dilemma, SERMs, rather than estrogen, may be your best choice.

My sister had a terrible time on HRT, especially the progesterone, and she quit HRT altogether. Does this mean that I'll be a poor candidate?

It's true that about 10 to 15 percent of women experience PMS-like symptoms from progesterone that are bad enough for them to want to stop taking the drug. Many of these symptoms clear up within five months. You don't say how long your sister waited before she stopped taking HRT. In any case, every woman is an individual when it comes to how she will respond to HRT, so it shouldn't matter.

Is there any danger to just stopping HRT, cold turkey?

No. The half-life of these medications is very short. But within days to weeks after coming off these medications, the effects of lack of estrogen will begin in terms of the heart, bones and cholesterol, and you will experience estrogen deprivation symptoms (i.e., hot flashes, dry vagina, etc.).

Do I run a greater risk of stroke by taking HRT?

The belief that hormone replacement therapy increases the risk of stroke is quite old and not adhered to any longer. It is similar to concerns about increased blood pressure. In the early days of hormone replacement therapy, it was felt that women with high blood pressure should not be offered estrogen because they were at great risk to develop stroke. This thinking has turned around 180 degrees. Now women with hypertension are among the first to be offered hormone replacement therapy because of the tremendous benefits that HRT can give the cardiovascular system in terms of reduction of heart disease and stroke.

Is it true that too much exercise lowers estrogen levels?

There are people who are exercise fanatics and have too little body fat, often accompanied by subtle or not-so-subtle forms of anorexia. Normal ovulation can be lost. Such women can develop what is known as hypothalamic hypogonadism, a medical term for losing your period and having low estrogen levels because there is insufficient output from the hypothalamus to tell the ovary to work. This isn't going to happen to you if you spend an hour at the gym each day.

Is it true that if you're a heavy coffee drinker—ten or more cups a day—you are at greater risk for osteoporosis?

Ten or more cups a day is truly pushing the limit. However, there is not strong scientific evidence that this is an accepted risk factor for osteoporosis. Certainly there have been concerns about excessive caffeine and its effect as a stimulant on the heart, blood pressure and even breast tissue. As a physician who sees all types of women day in and day out, my advice is to attempt moderation whether it is with caffeine or virtually anything else in your diet or lifestyle.

I'm forty-nine years old. My mother and father both have had heart attacks. Although my father died, my mother had angioplasty to unblock clogged arteries and is doing pretty well at eighty-four. None of my female relatives have had breast cancer, although an aunt had benign breast lumps that were removed in surgery. I worry about the breast cancer risk that I would have with HRT. How do I figure my risks and benefits and make the right choice?

I wish there were a numerical equation that I could give you to exactly balance risks and benefits, your fear of breast cancer versus your fear of heart disease. There isn't one. It certainly sounds like your family history is much stronger for heart disease than for any breast cancer. Your aunt's benign breast lumps don't really count as a family history of breast cancer. Currently the positive effect of estrogen on heart disease is fairly well established. If you have no trouble with traditional HRT, I would recommend that you use it for the time being. In the following chapters you'll learn how SERMs, especially Raloxifene, lower cardiovascular risk factors and why this might be a good choice for you in the future.

I took birth control pills from when I was nineteen up until about a year before I had my children in my thirties. Then I went on low-dose birth control pills because I was having heavy bleeding at all times of the month. Now at forty-nine, I am told I should switch to HRT because of night sweats that wake me sometimes three times a night. I've been hearing a lot about Raloxifene. It might be the right thing for me a couple of years from now, to prevent a heart attack or osteoporosis. But by taking all of this medicine, one pill after another, I'll have spent almost a lifetime on estrogen. Is this dangerous?

In the first place, if you're having night sweats while taking low-dose birth control pills, I suggest you have your doctor check your FSH level on day six of the pill-free (or placebo) week. If your FSH is elevated, then in fact you are menopausal and your doctor is correct in suggesting you switch to HRT. Realize, however, that the available active estrogen to your system on low-dose birth control pills is approximately double that of the standard starting dose for HRT. For example, 20 mcg of ethinyl estradiol in birth control pills such as Loestrin 1/20 or Alesse is equivalent to about 1.25 mg of Premarin.

Have you noted at what point in your cycle you're most uncomfortable? Does it seem to occur mostly in the one out of four weeks when you are on "dummy" pills? In my practice, patients who complain of symptoms on low-dose pills sometimes are having those symptoms in the one out of four weeks when they are not on medication. If this is true for you, you can try to shorten the pill-free interval by taking four weeks on and one week off or five weeks on and one week off. Even six weeks on and one week off can be effective. The manufacturers of birth control pills (for women like you, I prefer to call them "cycle regulators") did you no favor by making them in twenty-eight-day blocks so they would mimic your period. There is no reason why you need to have a withdrawal bleed thirteen lunar months in a calendar year. Six or seven withdrawal bleeds would be more than sufficient.

However, the crux of your question is whether women are endangered in some way by taking a lifetime of estrogen supplements or replacements. First of all, realize that for most of your lifetime you were making your own estrogen. Your breasts and your uterus were receiving a potent estrogenic message from the time you began having periods until a natural menopause would have taken place (average age 51.4). Strange as it may sound, if you nursed your children, you were in one of the most hypoestrogenic states at the time. By suppressing your own ovarian production of estrogen with low-dose birth control pills, the actual effective total amount that your breast would "see" is probably less than what you would make from your own body.

TWO

the SERMS *solution*

With 60 million women reaching menopause in the year 2000, and up to 80 percent of them turning away from conventional estrogen replacement therapy for fear of cancer, drug researchers everywhere have been asking the same questions: How can we create something for these women that has as many of the positive effects of estrogen while minimizing the negatives? Isn't there some way to customize estrogen?

A new category of drugs known as SERMs have shown promise. Scientists at every major drug company began working with them. Three years ago, one SERM, Raloxifene, developed by Eli Lilly, broke from the pack. The release of Raloxifene, under the trade name Evista, in January 1998 made the front pages of many of the nation's newspapers. For the first time, a SERM with an unparalleled record of safety was available. However, the FDA approved it only "for the prevention of osteoporosis in post-menopausal woman." Headlines in newspapers across the USA proclaimed it the "new osteoporosis drug." Chances are, if you weren't particularly worried about osteoporosis, you scanned these stories with little interest. After all, what did this have to do with your own dilemma about whether or not you should take HRT? Few newspapers were calling it the new HRT.

There is, however, a bigger story to tell. SERMs are probably the most potentially promising breakthrough in medicine for midlife women to have come along in the last two decades. In my opinion, the future for solving the estrogen dilemma is clearly going to be this cutting-edge category of drugs. Moreover, the risk of breast cancer and uterine cancer may be markedly diminished in your lifetime through SERMs. The ultimate potential may be estrogen customized for each woman's particular physical needs.

But today's available SERMs aren't miracle drugs. They don't presently do everything at menopause you might wish they would do. Your decision about whether and when to use them can be made with confidence, however, once you fully understand them.

What can selective estrogen presently do for your health? In this chapter you'll learn the following:

- SERMs solve the estrogen dilemma *by acting like estrogen where you need it*—in bone, lipid and probably heart—*but by acting like an antiestrogen where you don't want it*—the breast and the uterus.

- Raloxifene, the newest SERM to be released, prevents bone loss. Recall that women can lose as much as 20 percent of the skeleton in the five years after menopause. Not so with Raloxifene.

- Raloxifene significantly reduces the incidence of new-onset breast cancer. Three years' worth of data indicate a significant reduction in breast cancer in those women taking Raloxifene compared with those who take nothing. Contrast this with the 30 to 40 percent increase from being on long-term conventional HRT.

- It doesn't cause proliferation of the uterine lining like estrogen does. Therefore, not only does it not heighten uterine cancer risk but it also seems to diminish it.

- You won't be bothered with a period for the rest of your life, as you will be on drugs such as Premarin.

- You don't have to take progesterone with it—and deal with breast tenderness and mood swings.

- It lowers cholesterol and triglycerides, which means major benefits for your heart.

WHAT EXACTLY ARE SERMS?

SERMs are Selective Estrogen Receptor Modulators. People joke that this is a name only a scientist could love, but once you get past the vocabulary, it's a name for a class of drugs that makes perfect sense given what they do:

• **Selective:** They act only on certain areas or body parts. The SERM Raloxifene (Evista) binds to estrogen receptors in the bone and lipids, activating them. However, Raloxifene binds to, but does not activate, estrogen receptors in the breast and uterus. Therefore some tissues, such as bone and lipid, see SERMs as estrogen (what doctors call agonists) and other tissues see them as estrogen *antagonists* (an estrogen blocker, so to speak). Essentially you get an estrogen effect where you need it, and you block out such an effect where you don't want it.

• **Estrogen:** The naturally occurring female hormone that is produced by the follicles that develop in a woman's ovaries. As I discussed in the last chapter, estrogen does many healthful things for a woman's body that have nothing to do with reproduction.

The level of estrogen in the body plummets after menopause, when the ovaries no longer function as they did in your reproductive years. Today's women will have an unprecedented amount of "nonreproductive" years for the first time in history due to increased life expectancy. We're just starting to see the ramifications of being without estrogen for long periods of time.

• **Receptor:** A specific site in the cells of the body that can be turned on or off by a compound such as a drug or natural substance, be it SERM or estrogen. It is estimated that there are three hundred estrogen receptors in the female body. When receptors are turned on, particular actions or effects occur.

• **Modulator:** Something that acts to regulate and/or activate.

It may sound complicated, but at its most basic, Evista is a tablet you take once a day, every day. I'll discuss what makes a woman a good candidate for Raloxifene in the next chapter. However, keep in mind as you read what follows that Evista is a drug that protects women from the *silent* changes of estrogen loss that critically affect your health over time, not the "noisy" symptoms, such as hot flashes and vaginal dryness, that precede the so-called silent passage.

The Raloxifene trials involved more than 12,000 women aged forty-seven to seventy-five in more than twenty-five countries. Running initially for three years, various studies looked at various end points: spine fracture, breast cancer rate, mental acuity, heart attack, cholesterol, strokes, uterine bleeding, uterine precancers and cancers as well as side effects.

The studies were double blind, placebo controlled—the gold standard of science. That means no woman knew if she was taking Raloxifene or not. In fact, one-half to three-fourths of the women took various doses of Raloxifene. One fourth took a placebo. Sometimes one-fourth of the patients took estrogen.

The Raloxifene trials are ongoing. They will continue to test the drug's effect on such things as spine fracture and breast cancer rates, mental acuity, heart attacks, strokes, Alzheimer's disease and side effects.

Here's what we know after three years of testing:

WHAT THE STUDIES SHOW

• *Raloxifene and your bones:* Evista preserves bone mass and increases bone mineral density, preventing bone loss at the spine, hip and whole skeleton. At twenty-four months of testing, compared with the placebo, the average increase in bone mineral density with 60-mg daily of Raloxifene was 2.4 percent in the spine, 2.4 percent in the hip and 2.3 percent in the total body. Raloxifene is known as an antiresorptive, which means it blocks bone resorption—the process by which old bone is dissolved and eliminated. This leads to a higher level of circulating calcium as well as an increase in bone density. While Raloxifene patients saw an increase in bone density, those on placebo with calcium supplements suffered a 1 percent loss over the same amount of time.

Why this matters to you: Raloxifene kept women from losing bone and did it significantly when compared to placebos. The women in the study didn't have osteoporosis. They didn't need to gain bone. They just needed to preserve it, and Raloxifene did the job.

Although taking calcium, doing weight-bearing exercise, and taking vitamin D are key steps a woman can take to protect her bones, you will still lose bone mass once your body stops making estrogen, no matter how diligently you take these measures. These healthy choices have value but cannot totally prevent bone loss if you do not intervene with Raloxifene, estrogen or other medications. A menopausal woman can lose as much as 20 percent of her skeleton in the first five years after her periods cease. This of course creates more fragile, more easily fractured bones. Something you do every day, such as lifting a bag of groceries, can cause subtle fractures of the spine, once this degenerative process is at hand. Warding off osteoporosis is a major health goal when one considers that a woman's relative risk of hip fracture is equal to her combined risk of developing breast, uterine and ovarian cancers.

What else you should know:

• Raloxifene was approved for prevention of osteoporosis, not treatment, which is important for you to know if your doctor has already given you a diagnosis of osteoporosis. Prevention means maintaining or slightly increasing bone density, thus preventing the development of osteoporosis. Treatment means a medication actually reduces the rate of fractures in patients already with known osteoporosis.

The FDA will approve a drug for prevention of osteoporosis if the manufacturer does two things: (1) proves that it preserves bone mineral density in a statistically significant fashion; and (2) shows through bone biopsy that it does not distort bone architecture in an abnormal way. Raloxifene met both criteria.

The Raloxifene studies are continuing. For instance, as this book went to press, data were presented that showed Raloxifene also prevented fractures in women with known osteoporosis. Fractures were reduced by approximately 50 percent compared with women on placebos.

• The clinical studies showed that estrogen is still the best antiresorptive for your bones. It increases bone density by about 5 to 6 percent as compared to Raloxifene's 2 to 3 percent. Unlike estrogen, however, Raloxifene does not increase the risk of endometrial or breast cancers, as we'll see in a moment. Plus, if you haven't already lost bone, Raloxifene may be enough of what you need to prevent such loss in the future.

• Even if you have some bone loss already, this doesn't mean you're doomed to getting full-blown osteoporosis. You may never develop it. If you catch the degeneration early, you can begin a preventive regime.

• Fosamax, a nonhormonal osteoporosis preventive *and treatment* which many women currently take, is also an antiresorptive. Fosamax has been shown to block the production of bone-destroying osteoclasts. However, Fosamax is not an easy drug to take. You have to take it with eight ounces of plain water immediately after you awaken. Then you shouldn't lie down for at least half an hour afterward or eat or drink anything for another thirty minutes. This is to safeguard you from developing ulcers of the esophagus from an incompletely swallowed pill.

• The "placebo" group of women in the Raloxifene studies received calcium. The rate of loss of bone in this group was less than it was in the placebo group of the Fosamax study! This means that compared to doing nothing, calcium alone will slow the rate of bone loss, although these women still lost bone.

Your body does not manufacture calcium. Your body must get any calcium you need from outside sources. If you don't have enough calcium in your diet, your system breaks down bone in order to supply it. The take-home message is: Take your calcium! Fifteen hundred mg per day is optimal.

• When studies find that a woman builds 2, 3 or 4 percent of bone on a medication, be it a SERM or estrogen or something else, realize that this is within the first two years or so of taking the drug—after which, the rate of increase plateaus. You don't continue to build 4 percent a year, or you'd end up with bones of steel. You don't need to keep building bone, if you aren't losing bone.

• *Raloxifene and your cholesterol:* Evista lowers total cholesterol and low-density lipoprotein (LDL) cholesterol (the bad cholesterol) and does not change high-density lipoprotein (HDL) cholesterol (the good cholesterol) or triglycerides.

Why this matters to you:

Cholesterol is a type of saturated fat that travels through your bloodstream and becomes a risk factor for heart attacks because it can clog arteries. Of the two types of cholesterol, the LDL causes plaque by carrying cholesterol to the artery walls, where it becomes imbedded. HDL actually helps remove plaque and block LDL.

What else you should know:

• Estrogens will increase HDL, while Raloxifene does not.

• Triglyceride levels (another risk factor for heart disease) typically climb in women taking estrogen but do not seem to do so in women taking Raloxifene. Fibrinogen levels are not affected by estrogen, yet Raloxifene lowers them. Fibrinogen is involved in the process of blood clotting.

• Whether its effects on cholesterol will translate into fewer heart attacks is unclear. It is generally felt that these lipids, referred to as secondary markers of cardiovascular disease, account for about 25 to 50 percent of heart disease risk. With Raloxifene you will have protection at a level you can't get from your diet or exercise alone.

• *Raloxifene and your uterus:* Evista does not cause stimulation of the uterus or the endometrium.

Why this matters to you: For one thing, you won't have a monthly period from taking Raloxifene. And you won't have to take progesterone supplements with it (i.e., Provera—a drug many women find difficult to tolerate). But more important is the safeguard against uterine cancer.

Without getting too technical, your uterus is made up of muscle surrounding an endometrial layer, which is full of glands whose function it is to become receptive to the developing embryo. The whole reason for that lining in your body is to house a baby and then aid birth. Estrogen makes the lining thicken. When a woman ovulates, the ovarian follicle converts to what is known as the corpus luteum (that's Latin for "yellow body" because it looks yellow). It secretes progesterone, which encourages the growth of blood vessels and glands so that the uterus is prepared to receive a fertilized egg. When pregnancy does not ensue fourteen days after ovulation, you shed that entire buildup (i.e., your period). Now you're left with a very thin layer, and the process starts all over again.

When women become menopausal, they make little estrogen and clearly no progesterone, and there's no stimulation (growth) of that lining. It stays in a low, inactive, thin state. This "unstimulated" state is what doctors expect to find when they examine a postmenopausal woman who is not taking estrogen. Anything else is unusual and usually means you have to undergo some tests to see why.

When women take estrogen, they get the same proliferation they used to get in the first half of every menstrual cycle. They continue to get it their entire life, or as long as they stay on estrogen. If a ninety-year-old woman takes estrogen, it will cause her endometrial lining to grow and thicken.

Without progesterone, the endometrium will keep growing. An endometrium that is growing unchecked can lead to hyperplasia, a breeding ground for precancerous changes. This is why your doctor gives you progesterone (usually Provera) to take ten to fourteen days a month with estrogen, so you'll slough off this lining. This is what causes women after menopause to continue getting their "period."

Women who take Prempro, known as continuous-combined HRT, take a small amount of progesterone (medroxyprogesterone acetate, which is the generic form of Provera) every day, with estrogen (Premarin) every day.

None of this will happen with Raloxifene because it does not stimulate the endometrium. I was called upon to help design the definitive tests to look for any changes in the uterus in the Raloxifene studies because that is my area of expertise. After reviewing even the preliminary data, I am sure of one thing: Raloxifene does not cause precancerous changes in the endometrial lining of the uterus.

What else you should know:

• If you're currently taking Prempro, bear in mind that 31 to 35 percent of women on continuous-combined HRT during the

Raloxifene trials who were taking it didn't have an inactive endometrium. It was in fact proliferating. When I saw that number, I thought, "Wow," because doctors and patients as well have been under the impression that Prempro would prevent any proliferation. When these statistics came up at a worldwide advisory board on which I sit, several luminaries in the study of estrogen replacement therapy abroad said, "That's no surprise. You Americans don't use enough progesterone." In the U.S., Prempro was initally only 2.5 milligrams of MPA. In Europe, they routinely use 5 milligrams of MPA with the Premarin. Recently, Prempro 5 was released, which is 5 milligrams of MPA. It's worth looking into if you're currently taking Prempro.

In any case, the key to understanding the excitement about the Raloxifene study is that there was no proliferation. It's a pure estrogen blocker in the uterus.

• *Raloxifene and your breasts:* Women taking Raloxifene had no more breast tenderness or abnormalities on their mammograms than those taking a placebo. This is because Raloxifene does not stimulate the breast.

Why this matters to you: Here's that word *stimulate* again. In simpler terms, if a medication doesn't "stimulate" the breast, it doesn't cause cell division and proliferation (growth). Women in the trials who were taking Raloxifene did not complain of tenderness and pain in the breast. More important, there are data that show women on Raloxifene had a statistically lower risk of breast cancer than those on a placebo. Pooled data on more than 7,000 participants over a thirty-month period saw a significant reduction (58 to 78 percent) in the incidence of newly diagnosed breast cancer. (See chapter 7 for more details.)

Let's take a closer look at breast cancer for a moment, and why you don't want any more estrogen "stimulating" your breasts. Breast cancer begins in the lining of the milk ducts. Extra cells form in this lining. As they continue to increase, you have a condition known as hyperplasia, which basically means too many cells. These cells can become atypical. They look different from other breast cells as they multiply and begin to fill the duct. Sometimes, for reasons we don't understand fully, those cells will just stay there in the duct. But about 30 percent of the time they'll break out. They'll move to the surrounding fat and you'll be diagnosed with breast cancer. If they move from there to a blood vessel or a lymph node and move through the rest of the body, it is said that they have metastasized. That is the most serious stage of breast cancer, and it can be life threatening.

Why does someone with every risk factor in the world never develop it, and someone else with no risk factors end up with life-threatening cancer? When cells divide and grow, it's because of our genes. One theory says that a woman may have a faulty gene in the breast. It "minds its own business" so to speak for years, and then something nudges it or damages it and it begins to mutate, or grow and change.

The whole debate about breast cancer, in the most simple, layman's terms, comes down to this: Can a normal healthy breast cell become cancerous by introducing certain medications or foods into your body? Or is it just that some women already have cells that are susceptible to the process of change and cancerous growth that will manifest if they are stimulated by substances that nudge them over the line? No one knows. When you read about things that can "cause" or "lead to" breast cancer, you are usually hearing about things in the environment scientists believe cause mutated genes to grow. Estrogen is often mentioned as the worst culprit.

Recall that your body has been making estrogen naturally for years. One could conclude that if estrogen causes breast cancer, once you get to menopause, you're pretty much home free. Just don't take any more of it, and if you've come this far, you've got 100 percent protection. Wrong. Unfortunately it doesn't work that way. There are plenty of women who have never taken HRT and who have breast cancer.

But, if you do take unselective estrogens like Premarin, Estrace, Ogen or even phytoestrogens (unselective means it has nothing to block its effects anywhere in your body), will it nudge some unknown faulty cell you might have inherited into proliferating? That's the crucial question, and it is where none of the studies agree. Since we don't fully know the answer, or why it happens to some women and not to others, there are many women who decide not to take the risk of estrogen, no matter whether it could benefit other organs or not.

What else you should know: What we do know is that Raloxifene is an antiestrogen in the breast. It's going to block the effects on your breasts of any estrogen currently circulating in your body—and women still have some estrogen that doesn't come from the reproductive organs.

• *Raloxifene and menopausal symptoms:* Raloxifene is *not* a treatment for the symptoms of menopause that estrogen generally relieves: hot flashes and vaginal dryness.

Why this matters to you: If your primary reason for wanting a prescription for Raloxifene is that you are having distressing symptoms, Raloxifene may not help. Raloxifene hit its home run with the silent changes of menopause for those women who are looking for health maintenance, not relief of symptoms. The woman with severe hot flashes going through menopause is not going to be aided by Raloxifene. In studies, women on hormone replacement therapy had a 6 percent incidence of hot flashes. Women on a placebo had an 18 percent incidence of hot flashes. The women on Raloxifene had a 25 percent incidence of hot flashes. However, they tended to be mild and short-lived.

What else you should know:

• Women who reported hot flashes while on Raloxifene described them as "mild." When I tell patients who are thinking of going on Raloxifene that they may get some hot flashes, most say, "So?" Some say, "They weren't so bad the first time I went through them."

When you talk to the patients themselves, they don't seem all that fazed by the concept that a drug this beneficial to their overall vitality and long-term postmenopausal health might induce some transitory hot flashes. Still, there are some other patients whose interest in estrogen has to do with getting rid of nuisance symptoms, and they have priorities different from those who are more interested in overall health maintenance.

• For 85 percent of women, the more annoying symptoms of no longer making estrogen will stop within one year of their final period, regardless of what they do. The situation stabilizes. The mood, concentration, and sleep disturbances diminish because there are no longer any small fluctuations of estrogen. Hot flashes and night sweats subside. However, what does not go away are the problems of dry vagina and bone loss.

• Women in the Raloxifene trials were allowed to self-medicate with estrogen cream if they were bothered by vaginal dryness. Only about 2 percent of the Raloxifene group and 2 percent of the placebo group did so.

• This is not to say that there can't eventually be a SERM that does relieve hot flashes and other nuisance symptoms. Right now scientists are looking for SERMs that will help manage hot flashes and improve certain elements of cognitive function as well. New SERMs are being created and studied as this book goes to press. Some scientists believe that the true potential of SERMs is a medication that is programmed to a woman's particular physical symptoms. Men, too, might benefit, depending on the drugs' effect on the prostate gland.

• *Raloxifene and blood clots:* A few women taking Raloxifene developed blood clots in their legs.

Why this matters to you: Deep vein clots, if undetected, can lead to a clot in the lung.

What else you should know: The risk of deep vein clots known as DVT—deep vein thrombosis—is exactly the same for women on HRT. The message here is that Raloxifene acts like estrogen on the venous system. Although the risk is slight, it is important to be aware of this side effect and to take steps to avoid it. Women who will be immobilized for any reason, such as surgery, should discontinue Raloxifene or HRT if they're on it, seventy-two hours prior.

• *Raloxifene and leg cramps:* Leg cramps also occurred in about 5 percent of women on Raloxifene compared to 1.5 percent of those on a placebo.

Why this matters to you: Leg cramps, while not medically dangerous, can be uncomfortable. They don't, however, mean you are developing blood clots in your legs.

What else you should know: As with any medication, there is often a period of transition in which most of the side effects are noticed. Do women just learn to cope and ignore such symptoms, or do the symptoms disappear? As the testing goes on for Raloxifene, there will be answers to that question. In any case, if the idea of leg cramps bothers you, keep in mind that 95 percent of the women in the trials never experienced them.

A word about side effects and how they are reported: The FDA will list any side effects that more than 2 percent of women report. Remember, the study patients do not know what they are on (it is a blind study), and they see the study nurse every three to six months. Only the reported side effects that are significantly different from those of the placebo are felt to be due to the drug. In the case of Raloxifene, these are only hot flashes and leg cramps. There is, however, a list of side effects mentioned in the package insert for Evista. One, for example, is nausea. It says 8.8 percent of women on Evista reported nausea. Read closer and you'll see that 8.6 percent of women on the placebo reported nausea as well! It's not a significant difference, so don't be misled. You might think, "Hey, 8.8 percent of the women taking Evista got nauseated. That's one in twelve; I don't want to take it." But 8.6 percent, or one in twelve, of the women taking "dummy pills" reported experiencing nausea.

MAKING SENSE OF THE RALOXIFENE STUDIES

You're going to hear more and more about SERMs. As the data on Raloxifene continue to break, you will hear reports that may seem confusing or even conflicting. Let me clear up some of the major misconceptions I've already heard about Raloxifene:

Misconception 1: Raloxifene—and SERMs in general—are "Estrogen Lite." There is no way that this is Estrogen Lite. If Evista were merely Estrogen Lite it would do everything that estrogen does, but just not as much. For instance, it would be not as good for bone, or heart, but not quite as bad in the uterus or the breast. That's not how it works. Evista is estrogenic in bone and lipid, but totally opposite of estrogen in the uterus and the breast.

Beyond that, a preventive agent is no good if women do not take it. The main reason my patients do not start hormone replacement therapy is fear of breast cancer. The main reason that my patients who start HRT and do not continue it is vaginal bleeding and breast tenderness. Raloxifene isn't going to give you Breast Tenderness Lite or Vaginal Bleeding Lite. You aren't going to get either symptom. It isn't a smaller dose of Premarin. It's from an entirely different family of drugs.

Misconception 2: Raloxifene will cause hot flashes and dry vagina and all of the kinds of symptoms that women are trying to avoid when they go on estrogen in the first place. Raloxifene isn't going to "give you" those symptoms. If you have them, it's because of the depletion of estrogen in your body that occurs with menopause. What Raloxifene isn't going to do is take these symptoms away, as estrogen can.

Having said that, keep in mind that there is a big difference between women who go on hormone replacement therapy for treatment of severe menopausal/perimenopausal symptoms, including hot flashes, and women who are not having a problem with symptoms but are more concerned with long-term health maintenance (i.e., preventing the ravages of osteoporosis or heart disease). The best treatment for acute menopausal symptoms is traditional estrogen. However, women who can expect to spend 40 percent of their lives in a postmenopausal state are becoming increasingly concerned about extending their health with the benefits of estrogen in terms of bone preservation, heart disease prevention and improved lipids. At the same time, if a medication can reduce breast cancer and reduce uterine cancer and avoid breast tenderness and avoid uterine bleeding, this would be the best of both worlds.

Although the Raloxifene studies released data that reported 24 percent of the women in the studies experienced hot flashes, realize that this was part of blinded placebo-controlled trials. Women did not know if they were on SERMs, placebo or even estrogen. Anything they reported to the study nurse during the twenty-four months of study was recorded. Thus 24.6 percent of women reported some hot flashes, but the discontinuation rate for hot flashes was 1.7 percent. Thus the hot flashes are felt to be mild and short-lived.

Misconception 3: You can take Raloxifene to fend off the nuisance menopausal symptoms that bother you and then quit when you're past the point. It's the other way around. I will explain in the next chapter why women who had nuisance symptoms and turned to Premarin or some other form of HRT and found relief should stay with it for the time being. This is not the group of women who should immediately opt for Raloxifene. It may in fact be the other way around, for now, with this new SERM. Women can use conventional HRT to ward off the nuisance symptoms and then posibly switch to a SERM like Raloxifene after one or two years.

Misconception 4: Women doing well on HRT should still switch to SERMs immediately.

The question is how long to stay with HRT. There are women who will benefit from taking conventional forms of HRT for the years in which their symptoms are at their peak. I do not tell my patients who are doing well on HRT to switch now that Raloxifene is on the market. But the benefits of estrogen only accrue as long as you stay on it—ideally if you stay on it throughout your lifetime. For some women, this is when the potential for danger also occurs.

Misconception 5: Approval for Raloxifene was "rushed through the FDA." True, the FDA gave Raloxifene an expedited review, and why not? A drug with such potential benefits should not be held up bureaucratically. An expedited review does not mean that Raloxifene wasn't extensively tested.

QUESTIONS WOMEN ASK:

Why can't I take a little estrogen and a little Raloxifene to get the best of both worlds?

That's a question I also asked when I was under the impression that Raloxifene would cause some hot flashes. It was tempting to think that a small dose of estrogen might counterbalance the hot flashes; Raloxifene would protect the bones, uterus and breasts; and everything would be perfect. Not so. The problem is that both of these compounds compete for the same receptor sites. It is unclear how much estrogen it takes to undo the good effect of Raloxifene to the breast and uterus. Since the dose of Raloxifene is 60 mg and since a typical dose of estrogen is .625 mg, it is tempting to think that these two are equivalent in terms of receptor status but that's not necessarily so. What if it turns out to be a question of who's on first?

There are no data whatsoever on the effects of combining estrogen and Raloxifene. It could actually intensify hot flashes.

It might undo the breast and uterine effect. It could increase blood clotting. And of course, when one combines any medications, one often gets a "whole" much greater than the "sum of its parts." Until we know more, this is a strategy fraught with unknown risks or benefits.

How do these drugs really work? How is it possible that they can do one thing in one part of the body and something else in another part?

V. Craig Jordan, director of the breast cancer research program at Northwestern University Medical Center in Chicago, has been working with SERMs since the early seventies. In terms of how SERMs actually work in the body, he says, "This is the billion-dollar question that the pharmaceutical industry is trying to propose a solution to. There are three theories that scientists are working on at the moment. One theory is that the estrogen receptor is the same in all places, but there are other proteins, called co-activators, that make the genes get turned on so that the drug is seen as an estrogen at that particular site. Those 'helper' proteins are missing in other sites.

"Another theory is if the estrogen receptor is like a plug in a socket in the DNA, an antiestrogen like Raloxifene may change the shape of the plug, so it can turn on a gene by binding to a different site of the DNA.

"The third theory is that there's a different receptor. We now call the one that we know and loved for thirty years the alpha estrogen receptor. Scientists also now refer to a beta estrogen receptor. The theory with the beta estrogen receptor is that Raloxifene produces its estrogenlike effects because the beta receptor is located in some sites, not in other sites. So alpha receptors may only be in the breast, perhaps beta receptors are present in the bones, for example."

How can a woman be sure that Raloxifene is safe?

I believe you can be confident about the safety of Raloxifene for an important reason: *the extensive testing.* When I was asked for my expertise, I helped devise the testing protocol for Raloxifene that would ultimately prove that Raloxifene does not stimulate the uterus. It included a combination of biopsy, vaginal ultrasound (which basically involves placing a specially shaped ultrasound probe into the vagina to get a picture of the uterus) and fluid-enhanced sonohysterography, a procedure whereby a small amount of sterile saline solution is put into the uterine cavity through a tiny plastic catheter. The vaginal ultrasound exam is then conducted while saline is being infused. The detail is phenomenal: A doctor can see the uterine lining almost as if he or she were looking at it under a low-power microscope.

When Evista hit the market, the data from this study were still being collected and analyzed, and therefore had not been released yet; but the interim data from an earlier Canadian study were thorough enough to conclude that Raloxifene caused no stimulation of the endometrial lining and did not cause polyps. This was much of the basis for the FDA approval and labeling that it is, in fact, safe in the uterus. The definitive study of uterine safety that I helped design has been completed since then, and Raloxifene at various doses caused no stimulation of the uterine lining, meaning any proliferation, hyperplasia (precancer) or cancers. There was no polyp formation and there was no increase in the thickness of the endometrium as measured with transvaginal ultrasound and saline infusion sonohysterography. These results were corroborated by old-fashioned endometrial biopsy as well.

Still, wouldn't it be safer to wait awhile longer and see what happens as women begin to take Raloxifene? I don't know if I'm comfortable being the first kid on the block to try a new drug.

Many of my patients bring up this question about long-term safety. Remember that the studies are ongoing. If you are now contemplating taking a drug like Raloxifene, by the time you read this there will be at least three and a half years' worth of data. When you've been on it for two years, there will be five and a half years' worth of data and we will have better information on which to base long-term recommendations. If you go on it now, you are not committing yourself to taking it for the rest of your life.

The medication packaging says Raloxifene HCl. What does HCl stand for?

Hydrochloride salt. This is a binding substance commonly used to make compounds more stable.

What about ovarian tumors? Can Raloxifene cause them?

The FDA advisory panel discussed this in an open forum. Some data showed a small number of certain strains of mice used in studying Raloxifene developed some very unusual ovarian *stromal* tumors. (Stroma is the inner substance of the ovary.) Human beings develop mainly *epithelial* tumors. (Epithelial refers to the outer covering.) Drugs that cause a marked increase in luteinizing hormone, which is involved in ovulation, are capable of causing such tumors.

There is no such thing as a postmenopausal mouse. In premenopausal mice, some of these stromal tumors were discovered. However, no one is recommending Raloxifene to premenopausal women. In postmenopausal women, Raloxifene actually causes a *decrease* in luteinizing hormone. Tamoxifen has been around for twenty years and has almost 10 million women-use years (this unit indicates the number of women times the number of years they have used a certain drug) and no increase in ovarian cysts or ovarian tumors has been shown. There is no basis for any concern about Raloxifene increasing ovarian tumors unless perhaps you belong to a particular stain of premenopausal mice.

Will Raloxifene replace HRT?

At this stage of the study, I don't believe so. Only estrogen can solve hot flashes. My experience tells me that many women only seek medication for symptoms that are disrupting their lives and feel much less enthusiastic about taking a drug for preventive health. This may change as women age and become more aware of the challenges facing them in the future as they live the next thirty or forty years postmenopause. SERMs will offer a very attractive alternative to HRT.

My feeling is that until the randomized clinical trials currently ongoing show that Raloxifene or some other SERM reduces heart disease, women who are on HRT because of strong family histories of heart disease should continue their current regimen. If researchers can develop a SERM that can give women everything positive that estrogen does without the potential dangers, then yes, it could conceivably make conventional HRT a dinosaur.

The bottom line is, the decisions about HRT and which form may be best for a particular woman are complex and should be taken one patient at a time. In the next chapter I will help you find a framework for making *your* decision.

THREE

are SERMS *for you?*

Should you phone your physician tomorrow and ask about a prescription for Evista? Despite all the positive qualities of this SERM, unfortunately it isn't for every woman. Many of my patients have become interested in Raloxifene since the news about it was reported in the media. I have this advice for most women already on HRT: "Wait. Stay on HRT. Let's reevaluate in a year."

I also had more than forty patients on my "waiting list," who wanted to be phoned as soon as Raloxifene was released so that they could get a prescription. These women knew the pros and cons, and I knew they were ideal candidates.

How do doctors make the distinction between a good candidate for the new SERM and a woman who will be better served through other means? How can you make the distinction, so you can better discuss this option with your doctor? This chapter will help you answer the question "Is Raloxifene for me?"

WHO IS THE IDEAL CANDIDATE
FOR RALOXIFENE?

Most doctors agree that Raloxifene would be a very viable choice for women who are past menopause and have the following characteristics:

- You can not, should not or will not take estrogen.
- You don't have the vasomotor symptoms of menopause. You aren't suffering from bad hot flashes, night sweats or palpitations secondary to hot flashes, either because you are over them or you never really got them. If you do have these symptoms, they are mild enough not to be bothersome or able to be controlled by over-the-counter remedies.
- Avoiding breast cancer is your major concern, perhaps because of your family history, or just because you fear the disease.
- You want to prevent osteoporosis.
- You tried HRT, but you did very poorly. Perhaps you had a hard time with the progestin phase of HRT. Or, for whatever reason, after trying HRT over a period of time, you just couldn't tolerate it.

Let's look at these one at a time:

• You can not, would not or should not take estrogen. Perhaps you've shared your health history with your doctor and you've been told that you can't take estrogen, even if you want to. You're what I think of as the disenfranchised woman. For you it isn't a question of the pros and cons of HRT but the fact that you are simply not a candidate. Raloxifene gives you an entirely new option, and was, in fact, created for women like you.

• **If hot flashes or dryness of the vagina aren't things that trouble you particularly, you are a better candidate for Raloxifene than the woman who suffers badly from these symptoms.** There have been some reports that say Evista increases hot flashes. That's not exactly what occurred during the clinical trials. In the trials, 24 percent of the women taking Raloxifene, at some point during the two years of the study, reported some hot flashes versus 18 percent of the women taking the placebo. That doesn't mean that a woman who has hot flashes and begins taking Raloxifene will suddenly begin having more hot flashes.

It's my belief that Raloxifene may or may not be helpful to you, depending on the extent of your symptoms. I would encourage you to look at three things in making your decision: (1) the extent to which your symptoms are disruptive of your life, and, consequently, how great your willingness to take medication to combat them, (2) the length of time you've been menopausal and (3) whether or not you are a candidate for conventional HRT.

The two most frequent complaints women who've reached menopause come to their doctors for help with are still vaginal dryness and hot flashes. I've had many patients who have handled vaginal dryness successfully with lubricants like Replens or Astroglide or estrogen creams. These medications are soothing, but it's important to realize that they won't do anything for the gradual urogenital changes. For these, estrogen creams have been useful.

A relatively new option if you're concerned about dryness is Estring, which is a vaginal ring that can stay for up to three months in the vagina, where it releases pure estradiol. It doesn't get systemically absorbed so it can be useful potentially even in women with a history of breast cancer. My own patients who use it are very pleased with it. I have checked their blood levels to make sure that their estrogen remains in a menopausal range (i.e., that the estradiol in Estring is in fact not being absorbed systemically). I have yet to have a patient who has not maintained a menopausal range of estrogen while using Estring.

As far as hot flashes are concerned, even though these are thought of as the number-one nuisance of menopause, some women have very few of them. "It's not so terrible," a patient recently told me. "It's kind of a tropical thing. You get hot and sweaty, you flush, then it goes away. Not so bad when you know what it is."

Susan, a fifty-three-year-old teacher, smiles at that description and rolls her eyes. "Lucky her. How about twenty of those tropical breezes a day? Having your whole face turn red, so you can't hide it? Or waking up drenched in the night. My husband asked flatly, 'What the hell is this? Why is the bed wet?'

"I'm not one of the lucky ones. Do you know when I decided enough was enough? I was meeting some parents to discuss their son's miserable fourth-grade report card. From looking at the father's face, I knew it was going to be a difficult parent conference. My classroom is on the third floor, but this was no time for the stairs. We piled into the elevator and I was already feeling warm. The flash hit before we sat down to talk. I tried to bully myself through it. But there's no talking your body out of a hot flash. Thank God these were middle-aged parents. The father wouldn't meet my eyes—he suspected what it was. His wife definitely *knew*, and I have to hand it to her. She was mad about her son's report card and had come to make a case about that, but she took a look at what was happening and tried to make pleasant conversation. It was a ridiculous situation. Here I was dripping sweat, in big salty beads running from my forehead down to my waist. The three of

us sat there embarrassed, trying to talk about the kid's recent spelling tests, as if nothing odd was happening. This flash didn't quit. I finally said, 'Excuse me, I'd like to get one of your son's other teachers who has some very positive things to say in on this,' and flew out of the room. I collapsed into a chair in the vice principal's office. 'Do you have any Kleenex?' I panted. She took one look at me and knew. I grabbed the box she handed me and started toweling myself off.

"I went back to that meeting and got through it, but something had changed for me. I knew I couldn't handle these symptoms anymore with a Tylenol or some deep breathing. And how is one supposed to do that anyway, in the middle of a parent conference? Imagine my saying, 'Excuse me, folks, I have to meditate now and hold this breath for the next sixty seconds then breathe out so I can stop this wave of heat coursing through my body. Afterwards we'll talk about your child's missing homework assignments.' It was impossible. Hot flashes were turning my professional life and any respect I had gained upside down."

Raloxifene isn't going to help Susan with her hot flashes. The best record for dealing with this symptom still belongs to conventional HRT. Susan rated her discomfort with her symptoms a nine out of ten. It was high enough for her to seek medical help.

Which brings us to the next point: If you are having bad symptoms, how far are you into menopause? Women think of menopause as being the prime time for unusual symptoms that interfere with their sense of well-being. But it's the decade before menopause, and especially the immediate months before your menstrual periods come to an end, that are the most disruptive. For many women, once menstruation stops, the difficult symptoms are soon over. They will end in a year or so, no matter what women do.

• **Are you concerned enough about preventing osteoporosis to take daily medication when you don't have the disease?** Many women aren't as concerned as they might be if they had the facts. *Prevention* magazine's June 1998 issue printed the results of a *Prevention*/NBC *Today Weekend* edition of their Pulse of America Survey, which is based on telephone interviews with women across the USA. Only 25 percent of women age fifty and over said that they saw osteoporosis as a very likely threat. Yet 50 percent of these women will break a bone because of this disease if you consider the current statistics. The survey also found that 69 percent of Americans don't take calcium supplements, and that only 26 percent of the at-risk group ever heard their doctors recommend a bone density test.

Who's at risk for osteoporosis? Here are the generally accepted risk factors in the form of questions you can ask yourself to judge your level of risk:

• Are you Caucasian or Asian?

• Have there been broken bones or stooped posture in older members of your family, especially women?

• Have you had a complete hysterectomy (ovaries removed also) but decided not to take estrogen?

• Is your diet low in calcium?

• Do you get little or no exercise?

• Has a close member of your family—your mother, grandmother, sister—been diagnosed with osteoporosis?

• Have you broken a bone recently? Did it happen from a mild accident, such as falling off balance versus something like skiing?

- Do you have a history of thyroid disease? Have you been diagnosed with hyperthyroidism, an overactive thyroid?
- Did you ever "miss" your period for more than six months when you weren't pregnant? Were you underweight, for example, or under stress?
- Do you smoke cigarettes?
- Do you have fair skin?
- Are you small boned, or do you think of yourself as "naturally thin."
- Have you ever used cortisone or antiseizure drugs, which can cause significant bone loss?

The more "yes" answers, the higher the degree of your risk. How can a woman find out the current state of her bones without the guesswork? The DEXA test has been used in the last decade to diagnose osteoporosis and its precursor, osteopenia (low bone mass). DEXA stands for dual-energy X-ray absorbitometry. It measures bone at the hip, spine and wrists, where most osteoporosis-related fractures happen. A DEXA test costs about $200, and is painless and quick. You lie fully clothed on an examining table for about twenty minutes while a scanner that emits low levels of X-ray radiation passes over you. Your results are compared to peak bone density for young adults, to show how much bone density you might have lost, as well as to that of your own age group. Results come in the form of a T-score. A T-score up to -1.0 is considered normal. A T-score between -1.0 and -2.5 is considered osteopenia, which means low bone mass, but not yet osteoporosis. A T-score less than -2.5 indicates osteoporosis.

While the DEXA test has been widely used, recently the U.S. Food and Drug Administration (FDA) approved a new device that uses high-frequency sound waves to measure bone density in the foot. Fast, easy and inexpensive, it's a device to measure the speed of sound and the attenuation of sound through the heel. You put your bare foot into a boxlike device, and the mechanism uses ultrasound to get a measure of the density and architecture of your heel bone. The faster the waves move through your heel bone, the healthier the bone. The entire test is painless and takes about ten seconds.

One might wonder how a device that looks at bone in your heel could tell you about your risks for a hip fracture. It works because all bones of the skeleton will reflect osteoporosis to some extent, and the heel is easiest to scan. While it is not as precise as a standard DEXA test, it can give you an idea of whether you actually need further testing.

• **Do you have a major concern about breast cancer? Raloxifene can give you significant prevention.** Women who have major risk factors for breast cancer have always found the decision about HRT frustrating. As I've said before, I believe that estrogen, at least in long-term use in postmenopausal women, is a promoter of breast cancer—not an inducer or cause. To use a metaphor, if there is a spark there, estrogen may ignite it. But estrogen doesn't create the spark.

The risk factors for breast cancer most doctors agree on include having had a female relative diagnosed with the disease, early menstruation (before age twelve), late menopause (after fifty-five), having no children or the first child after thirty, heavy alcohol consumption and obesity. However, there are studies that show that most women with these known risk factors never develop the disease. Remember that risk factors are behaviors or traits that increase your chances of getting a disease, but they are derived from groups of people, not individuals. Risk factors also have a cumulative effect. You should therefore do what you can to eliminate risk factors you have within your control, such as losing weight if you need to, etc.

The good news is that two studies confirm that Raloxifene can reduce the incidence of breast cancer by as much as 74 percent. One study, directed by Dr. Steven Cummings of the University of California at San Francisco, followed 7,705 postmenopausal women with osteoporosis for thirty-three months. Those taking Raloxifene showed a 74 percent reduction in the incidence of breast cancer.

A second study, directed by Dr. Craig Jordan of Northwestern University, pooled data from 10,553 women ages forty-one to eighty, which is significant because the sample included women who were younger and not suffering from osteoporosis, unlike the Cummings study. Jordan found a 58 percent overall reduction in breast cancer among those on Raloxifene.

• **Are you a woman who tried HRT and couldn't tolerate it?**
Alice, forty-nine, remembers, "My body just wouldn't tolerate Provera. My doctor suggested I try some different variations, but my heart wasn't in it. I was never that sold on HRT to begin with. I was scared of breast cancer."

Raloxifene becomes an exciting new option for women like Alice who otherwise will spend one-third of their lives in a low-estrogen state. More than 80 percent of women who are prescribed HRT discontinue it within two years, so there are many, many women who fall into this category. If Alice doesn't have any factors in her health history that would preclude her taking Raloxifene—venous thrombosis, for example—she's an excellent candidate because she's ruled out the best competing option.

In my own practice, the women who went on Evista as soon as it became available were women who had been on nothing before because of fear of breast cancer, but knew they were at risk for heart disease and osteoporosis. Some were women who were reluctantly on HRT because of family histories of these illnesses, but still had a great fear of breast cancer and wanted to get off estrogen as soon as something else was available.

COULD RALOXIFENE STILL BE RIGHT FOR YOU?

Every woman's health history is different. Perhaps you do not fit the profile for the ideal candidate for Raloxifene. Could it still work for you? Here are some common scenarios:

• **What if you still menstruate, but only sporadically?** I'd define menopause as not having a menstrual cycle for six consecutive months, given that one is the appropriate age. I've had patients who are fifty-plus, have no period for four months, conclude "This is it" and then end up resuming menstrual cycles again. This is because the ovary function doesn't succumb in one fell swoop. It often sputters. Women who are not definitely in menopause are poor candidates for Raloxifene. It seems unlikely, but they could get pregnant if they still ovulate, and Raloxifene could be dangerous to the fetus. And there are better treatments for a woman who is approaching menopause—for example, low-dose birth control pills such as Loestrin 1/20 or Alesse.

Leigh, forty-nine, hadn't had a period for three months. "I figured, this was menopause. But I was dressing to go out to dinner one evening when I saw I was spotting. I'd been planning to wear new white slacks and nothing else in the closet zipped, I was so bloated.

"I spotted for two more days. Saturday morning I woke up to a deluge. I ran to the bathroom twenty times that day to check my clothes. I finally ditched the tampons and bought the first batch of maxi pads I'd had in years.

"I felt sick and listless and fat. Two more days of the crimson tide, then nothing. Five days of spotting followed and I was sick and tired of all this bleeding. It was the longest, grossest, weirdest cycle I've ever had, and I wanted to know why I had it. That was about forty days ago, and I haven't had any bleeding since, thank the Lord for small favors."

Having heard this scenario scores of times from patients, I had a feeling that what Leigh was experiencing wasn't menopause, but perimenopause, the transitional period women go through just prior to the cessation of their menstrual cycle. During perimenopause the body is still producing estrogen, but women are no longer ovulating each month.

Leigh wanted blood tests to confirm what was happening. I gave her a test for the level of estradiol (a form of estrogen) in her blood and for FSH (follicle stimulating hormone) level. FSH is the hormone that stimulates the egg in the ovary. Its level becomes high for women who are postmenopausal. The pituitary gland makes FSH to signal the ovary to function. When the ovary cannot respond because there are no eggs, more and more FSH is pumped out to try to stimulate the ovary to respond.

Her blood tests gave contradictory results. She had premenopausal levels of estradiol in her blood, but her FSH levels had started to rise. Given laboratory norms, her estrogen levels showed her to be premenopausal while her FSH levels showed her to be postmenopausal.

It's a classic case of what happens to a woman's body during perimenopause, a developmental stage prior to menopause, when such strange on-and-off cycles of bleeding can occur along with some more subtle symptoms such as forgetfulness, insomnia, anxiety and mood swings. These symptoms can be so subtle and confusing that women don't relate them at first to their changing menstrual pattern. Since the stage of perimenopause can last as long as a decade, some women find themselves at the psychiatrist before they get to the gynecologist.

What causes the symptoms of perimenopause? When a woman doesn't ovulate—and this is a frequent fact during perimenopause—her body produces estrogen but she doesn't produce any progesterone; it is only with ovulation that an ovary will produce progesterone. Progesterone and estrogen work together to create a hormonal balance. When there is no progesterone production, estrogen is said to be unopposed. Unopposed and often fluctuating levels of estrogen circulating in the body cause these discomfitting symptoms.

Hormonally speaking, what's regular for a woman in transition is irregularity. This is why it's important that you get more than just a single FSH test to confirm menopause. If FSH is the only thing that is being tested, and the reading is high, a doctor might conclude that you are menopausal and recommend hormone replacement therapy when it isn't necessary yet.

I have seen numerous patients whose blood tests were in the menopausal range, and then they subsequently had a last episode of ovarian function, produced some estrogen, had some bleeding, and a new test showed them to be in a premenopausal range.

Leigh was interested in Raloxifene, but it isn't for women like her. If you are still menstruating, even very sporadically, Raloxifene is not an option. For one thing, you can still get pregnant if you do occasionally ovulate, and Raloxifene could be harmful to the developing fetus. Second, Raloxifene isn't going to be effective with any of your perimenopausal symptoms. But most important, it hasn't been tested in premenopausal women and it's not clear what it will do in premenopausal women. There are really no data, and I therefore wouldn't give it to a woman who wasn't clearly in menopause. There's no proof of efficacy, and the side effects could be very different. In the laboratory mouse, for example, a mammal that is always premenopausal, you get markedly elevated levels of LH (luteinizing hormone) whereas in postmenopausal women there is a decrease in LH with Raloxifene. In premenopausal women it might very well cause an increase in LH and act like a very different drug.

What kind of help is available for Leigh, close to menopause but not really there yet? I recommend low-dose birth control pills. Today this is the most effective treatment for perimenopausal symptoms. Don't let "birth control" throw you. I tell my patients who have found relief from the new low-dose birth control pills to look at them as "cycle regulators." Today's low-dose pills such as Loestrin 1/20 and Alesse do not carry the risk of stroke and heart attack which were dire warnings for women over thirty-five taking the pill in the 1970s. They consist of combinations of very low amounts of estrogen and different progesterones. They work by turning off the ovary's natural estrogen production and substituting it with a measured amount of estrogen and progesterone all month long—actually less than your body would make normally. These pills eliminate the symptoms caused by fluctuating levels of unopposed estrogen. In addition, today's low-dose oral contraceptives provide the following protections:

- protection against ovarian and endometrial cancer
- less breast disease
- fewer ectoptic pregnancies
- less iron-deficiency anemia
- less pelvic inflammatory disease (PID)

- less rheumatoid arthritis
- increased bone density

• *What if your biggest concern is avoiding heart disease?*

Grace at fifty-four was definitely postmenopausal. She told me this: "My grandmother had a heart attack at age seventy. It happened so fast, no one even had time to call the paramedics. She grabbed her chest, said she felt sick, sank down on her bed and it was over. My father, who was about fifty pounds overweight, collapsed on the stairs on the way to his bedroom after coming home from work one night and was dead minutes later. He was fifty-nine. Now that I'm in my fifties, I'm very concerned about heart disease."

It's true that all human beings past the age of fifty are at some risk for heart disease. Postmenopausal women are more vulnerable to heart disease because they no longer have estrogen's positive effects on blood cholesterol levels unless they take estrogen supplements.

For women whose biggest concern is avoiding heart disease, I still recommend estrogen over Raloxifene. The definitive studies on Raloxifene's direct effect on the heart are ongoing. Although Raloxifene does have a positive effect on the lipids, estrogen has a longer track record of improving cardiac health.

Which factors increase your risk of heart disease?
- having diabetes
- having a parent who had a heart attack before age sixty-one
- high blood cholesterol (greater than 200 milligrams) and/or HDL (good cholesterol) lower than 35 milligrams
- high blood pressure

- smoking cigarettes
- drinking more than three alcoholic beverages daily
- being an African-American
- being physically inactive
- stress

Eli Lilly has begun a large study to determine if Evista can prevent heart attacks or heart disease. The Raloxifene Use for the Heart (RUTH) trials began enrolling 10,000 women at risk of heart attack worldwide in May 1998. The trial will last up to seven and a half years.

• **What if you have osteoporosis?** During the Raloxifene trials, the scientists checked women's bones by measuring bone mineral density. They found that women taking Raloxifene had upped their bone density by an average of 2 to 3 percent, while those taking the placebo had lost bone. Still, if you already have osteoporosis, or skeletal fractures, there are other agents approved for *treatment*, not prevention, including Fosamax and Calcitonin. As a result of newly released studies, we can look forward to Evista being approved soon for the treatment of osteoporosis as well.

• **What if you've had breast cancer?** Let's say you currently have breast cancer. Tamoxifen (also a SERM and a cousin of Raloxifene, which I will talk about in depth in chapter 7) has 10 million women-use years as adjuvent chemotherapy for women with newly diagnosed breast cancer. Tamoxifen attaches to estrogen receptors and competes with a woman's own natural estrogen for these receptor sites. In the breast, Tamoxifen blocks the receptor sites, thereby preventing cancer cells from dividing. But the problem with Tamoxifen is that it can stimulate estrogen receptors in the endometrial lining, causing cell growth and increasing the risk of uterine cancer. Raloxifene was pursued because it lacks this dangerous effect. You can, however, monitor this side effect through gynecological ultrasound examinations and saline infusion sonohysterography.

Clearly Tamoxifen is still the drug to go on if you have recently diagnosed breast cancer. If you have finished five years of Tamoxifen, the National Cancer Institute recommends that you come off, although many of my patients in the past have elected to stay on if they've encountered no proliferation of the endometrium (a side effect of Tamoxifen which can be dangerous). This was because Tamoxifen was their form of hormone replacement therapy in that it lowered cholesterol and protected their bones. Now if you're a woman who comes off of Tamoxifen in five years, what do you do? You can do nothing more, of course. You can go on estrogen—which none of the women in my practice seem willing to do because of the fear that estrogen will cause a recurrence of breast cancer. You can continue Tamoxifen, which isn't recommended by the National Cancer Institute. Or, you can go on a SERM such as Raloxifene. Although it has not been specifically studied in women like you, based on everything I understand, if you're a woman who has finished your five years of Tamoxifen, that would be your best choice.

You may feel like one of my patients, Mary, who has been on Tamoxifen for seven years after a bout with breast cancer. "It was risky to go two more years, when five years on Tamoxifen is supposed to be the max, but after long talks with my doctor, I went ahead. But, after seven years, it was just like going into the land of the unknown. I didn't know what to do at this point. I didn't like being without Tamoxifen. I honestly thought of having a hysterectomy. My thinking was if I remove my uterus and ovaries, I can eliminate all risk of one of the two cancers I'm worried about.

But, that, of course, is major surgery. Still, once you have a scare with cancer, you get a little more drastic about what you'll try not to have that worry again, I think. Until Raloxifene, I felt like I really didn't have an option." Mary is on her fourth month of Raloxifene and relieved as even more promising data about the drug are released.

• *What if you're concerned about Alzheimer's disease?* The trouble is, we simply don't know enough about what causes Alzheimer's disease yet. Here's what we do know: Four million Americans now have the disease. It is more widespread now because more people are living past the age of sixty-five, which is the age range in which 90 percent of the cases occur. It's slightly more common in women than men, basically because women still tend to live longer. What are the risks once you reach your senior years? About 10 percent at age sixty-five, 20 percent at age seventy-five and 40 percent at age eighty-five. If you have close relatives who have acquired the disease, you are more likely to get it because you may also have a gene—the apoE gene on chromosome 19, more commonly called apoE4—which roughly half of Alzheimer's victims carry and researchers believe may be the culprit. Although you can be tested to see if you carry this gene, it's hardly worth it, in my opinion. Half of Alzheimer's sufferers don't have it, and if you do find you have it, your fears can be raised unnecessarily, and you can only do what all of us should do—take the health measures you can to avoid the disease. If you don't have the gene, it's not an all-clear signal. You still can acquire Alzheimer's.

If you've stopped being able to recall phone numbers and you keep misplacing your keys, should you worry that you have the disease? Not necessarily. The problem is when you forget what the keys are used for! Forgetfulness is one of the primary subtle symptoms women endure once their body stops making estrogen and progesterone naturally in the decade before menopause. It often disappears once a woman's body reaches menopause. Memory loss is also common in all people as they age. I can also assure you that I've known many patients who feared Alzheimer's when they were suffering from medication side effects, thyroid problems and infections.

There are no drugs that are currently approved by the FDA to *prevent* the disease. However, three of four large studies in the last decade suggest that women who take estrogen may get some protection, or delay the onset of the disease. One study done at a California retirement home showed estrogen users to have 50 percent less risk than nonusers. Researchers in Baltimore and New York found that estrogen reduced risk by 54 percent and 87 percent, respectively. The bottom line for my patients is this: If you are concerned about Alzheimer's and have a strong family history, my first suggestion to you would not be Raloxifene but conventional estrogen replacement therapy. Research is going on right now as to how Raloxifene interacts with brain tissue. Soon we will know whether it acts like estrogen in the brain. If it does, it may be helpful in the prevention of Alzheimer's.

• *What if what you're looking for is something to make you feel better?* Raloxifene is preventive medication. It does not necessarily make women feel any different while they are taking it. There's also no evidence that it won't make you feel better.

If you're feeling bad because of hot flashes, night sweats, insomnia or moodiness, Raloxifene is not designed to help and does not have the track record estrogen has. Estrogen replacement reduces the number of hot flashes, usually within one to three months. There is no evidence that Raloxifene will have a negative effect on sleep habits or patterns, but there is no evidence that it will improve them either. Many women have reported a "tonic" effect taking HRT, but it's always been unclear if it was the estrogen affecting the mood or the relief from symptoms.

• **What if you've been on HRT for more than five years?** You may well want to consider switching to Raloxifene, depending, of course, on the other factors in your health history and on your goal for taking HRT. If you were taking HRT to relieve menopausal symptoms, chances are you are well enough past the initial uncomfortable period of menopause to make estrogen use for that purpose no longer necessary. If preventing osteoporosis and breast cancer is your goal, you may want to explore Raloxifene. I predict that many women will take traditional HRT in the twelve to eighteen months of the transitional stage when their symptoms are bothersome. However, once that phase is over, I think women will make the transition to a SERM product for health maintenance for the long term.

What if you've been taking estrogen for more than ten years? You may seriously consider switching. This is when cancer risks may start to rise.

MAKING YOUR DECISION

If you find that you're a good candidate for Raloxifene, what else might you consider before you see your doctor?

This brief questionnaire can help confirm your decision. Read the questions below and choose the answer that comes closest to what's truest for you:

1. How often do you see your gynecologist?
   a. Twice a year.
   b. Once a year.

c. When I'm having a problem.

d. It's been several years, I think.

2. When did you last have a mammogram?

a. Within the past year.

b. Within the past two years.

c. Two or more years ago.

d. I have never had a mammogram.

3. Which of the following statements is true about your cholesterol?

a. I know my cholesterol levels and they are in an acceptable range.

b. I know my cholesterol levels and they are higher than I'd like them to be.

c. I don't know my cholesterol levels, but I'm sure I've been tested.

d. To my knowledge, I haven't ever had my cholesterol tested.

4. When you are taking a prescription drug, which statement is most true about you?

a. I take it steadily as directed and have a discussion with my doctor if I want to stop.

b. I sometimes get so busy I forget to take it or refill it.

c. I rarely take prescription drugs.

d. I avoid all medications and prefer to treat myself with diet or herbal remedies.

5. The prospect of taking a pill each day indefinitely

a. Doesn't bother me if it will help protect me from illness.

b. Bothers me a little, but I guess I'd do it if I thought I would benefit.

c. Bothers me a great deal, and I think I'd resent it.

d. I would never do it, for any reason, unless it was keeping me alive.

6. If I got mild leg cramps or hot flashes from medication

a. It wouldn't be the end of the world; I could deal with it if there was a benefit in exchange.

b. I might stop taking the medication if they were bad.

c. I would definitely stop taking medication that brought on leg cramps or hot flashes, however mild. I take medication to feel better, not worse.

d. I wouldn't even try a medication that could have these things as a side effect.

7. How do you feel about taking conventional HRT (hormone replacement therapy)?

a. I either can not, will not or should not take estrogen.

b. There's nothing in my family history to prevent me from taking it, but I fear increasing my risks of breast cancer.

c. I'm currently on HRT, but I'm not fully convinced that it's the right decision.

d. I'm doing great on HRT and I've been on it for more than five years.

8. If you were given a prescription for a drug that had only been on the market a year, how would you feel?

a. Fine with it, if my doctor is fine with it.

b. Concerned enough to do a lot of reading about it.

c. Very concerned; I would probably not take it.

d. Totally concerned. I would worry that down the road the drug causes problems no matter how convincing the testing of the drug was.

9. **If your doctor recommended Raloxifene and you found your health insurance did not cover it, how would that influence your decision?**
   a. It wouldn't matter to me, if I thought I should be on it. My health is worth spending money on, so whether or not my health insurance covers something isn't the sole deciding factor for me.
   b. I would have mixed feelings about taking it, especially if the policy *did* cover HRT, but I wouldn't rule it out completely.
   c. I wouldn't or couldn't fill a prescription that wasn't covered on my health plan.
   d. I do not have health insurance, and medical bills are a burden for me.

10. **Think about the last prescription drug you took. Which of the following statements is most true for you?**
    a. I was well aware of the side effects of taking it and knew what to look for.
    b. I didn't really know the side effects, but if I get ill taking a drug, I call my doctor.
    c. I was taken by surprise to hear that there were side effects after I had been taking it awhile.
    d. I don't like to know about side effects, because then I either become afraid to take the drug or think I'm having every side effect in the book.

11. **If you were taking a prescription drug and couldn't tell that it was having any effect on you, what would you be most likely to think?**
    a. "So what? I don't have to feel something to know that it is working."
    b. "Is it working? Is it worth it?"

c. "Why am I paying money for this, if it doesn't make me feel any better?"

d. "Forget this. I only take prescription drugs for very serious symptoms, and they have to work fast or I stop taking them."

12. What are your health goals now that you've reached menopause?

a. To maintain my health and prevent future health problems that could occur now that my body is no longer creating estrogen.

b. To prevent future problems of which I have a serious family history with medication if necessary; I don't worry about the rest.

c. To handle menopause in a natural way.

d. I'm not sure of my goals and don't generally waste time thinking too much about the future.

WHAT YOUR ANSWERS MEAN:

Mostly A's: If your doctor recommends Raloxifene, you will probably find it easy to take and be very happy with your choice. You are probably more interested in prevention and maintenance of your health at this moment than in ridding yourself of symptoms. That's what Raloxifene is all about.

Mostly B's and C's: Your feelings about SERMs are probably mixed. You have somewhat negative feelings about taking medication for prevention, and you wonder if the benefit is worth the risks, the money, and the effort. Reading the rest of this book might help make your decision clearer, as would a frank discussion with your doctor.

Mostly D's: Even though you might be offered SERMs, you probably won't consider them seriously, and/or have a difficult time maintaining your motivation to take them. You may be struggling with symptoms. You may have misgivings about synthetic drugs or new technology. The rest of this book will either allay those suspicions or at least give you information you should have to confirm your choice.

HOW TO ANALYZE YOUR ANSWERS

Why do A answers indicate that SERMs are probably right for you? Here are my thoughts on each of the questions.

1. It's important when beginning a new medication that you follow up with regular checkups. I see my patients twice a year. The more often one screens, the fewer things fall through the cracks. I can't prevent bad things from happening, but increased surveillance is likely to yield earlier detection. It also gives me a chance to reevaluate my patients' status in terms of health, family histories and medications they are considering taking. Things are happening relatively quickly. A year is a long time.

2. Every woman who has reached menopause should have regular annual mammograms. Beyond the health sense this makes, and the peace of mind you can achieve, such a step shows that you are committed to protecting your health. That kind of thinking makes you a good candidate for drugs like Raloxifene, which are, after all, about protection rather than relief.

3. As a secondary marker of coronary heart disease, the level of your cholesterol is important to know. Don't assume it's low because you feel fine. You also want to know your levels before you decide between estrogen and Raloxifene. If your levels are very high, then there are drugs that are specific for lipid lowering that are more potent. If your levels are only slightly elevated or normal, then you are a better candidate for Raloxifene. Remember, it lowers cholesterol about 12 percent, so if that is going to be enough for you and your doctor to feel confident, then it's a good choice. If you need more than that you may require a specific lipid-lowering medication.

4. A preventive drug is no good if you do not take it. Raloxifene must be taken daily and steadily to have its positive effect. This has always been a problem with HRT. Women take it when their symptoms bother them, and then drop it a year or so later. That strategy does nothing to fend off osteoporosis or heart disease. The best benefits accrue over time.

5. There is probably no such thing as taking enough Raloxifene so that you can stop one day and be protected from osteoporosis for life. It appears you need to continue taking it for as long as you want prevention. Still, does this mean the rest of your life?

What I tell patients is that I recommend embarking on a five-year plan. I am confident that well within that five-year time frame, there will be additional information allowing you to fine-tune your plans to continue or not. If you are contemplating taking a drug like Raloxifene, by the time you read this there will be at least three and a half years' worth of data. That means when you've been on it for two years there will be at least five and a half years' worth of data and better information with which doctors can make long-term recommendations. If you go on it now, you are not committing yourself to doing it for the rest of your life.

6. Symptoms of leg cramps and/or hot flashes reported during the Raloxifene trials were so mild that they did not cause many women to drop out of the study. However, if you do decide to take Raloxifene, you have to be aware that this could happen to you in the first few months. Generally, it's not a problem after that.

7. Women who are happy with HRT and doing well on it should stay with it for the time being, in my opinion. Raloxifene is the best choice for women who will not take estrogen, or have tried HRT and have not done well. Otherwise, their only other option is to live with a low estrogen state and try to ameliorate symptoms and disease through diet and exercise, which might very well not be enough.

8. If you were to fill a prescription for Raloxifene tomorrow, there would be three and a half years of existing data out there to back up your choice. Women who feel that a drug must be on the market for years before they are comfortable taking it aren't going to be happy with SERMs.

9. Raloxifene costs roughly $65 per month. Yes, HRT is cheaper, running about $40 a month for prescriptions for Premarin and Provera. As far as whether your insurance will cover it is concerned, as this book went to press, Raloxifene was FDA approved only for the prevention of osteoporosis. If that is why your doctor is prescribing it, indications are that most plans will cover it.

10. Although there are very few side effects with Raloxifene, I believe women should know what they are up front and monitor themselves carefully. While it's true that knowing there are side effects can make anyone a little anxious, there is no greater anxiety than not knowing and thinking something is seriously wrong with you when you experience a side effect.

11. You probably aren't going to "feel" anything on Raloxifene. You might feel that sense of well-being often reported with estrogen. If you don't, the way you can be assured that it is working is possibly having your bone density tested if you've already had it done, and comparing the figures. If you feel you have to "see" or "feel" results to maintain your motivation to take a drug, you may well not be happy with Raloxifene.

12. Women who opt for SERMs are generally more interested in health maintenance than curing menopausal symptoms. They are also highly motivated to protect their health—you'd have to be to invest in a drug you take daily, for years.

QUESTIONS WOMEN ASK

Why can't they invent a SERM that does it all?

Believe me, every major drug manufacturer is very interested in doing just that. In the last chapter of this book you can read about the progress of the other SERMs that are in the trial stages. I don't think that a SERM that does it all is out of the question in your lifetime.

If I take Raloxifene, do I still have to do weight-bearing exercise?

You will get twice the benefit if you do. Remember that weight-bearing exercise helps one maintain flexibility as well as strength. You don't want to be a woman who can't bend down to pick up her grandchild, or get out of the back seat of a taxi.

I gained weight, big time, on Prempro—forty pounds. Will I gain weight on Raloxifene?

There is no evidence that Raloxifene or any of the SERMs results in any weight gain. Certainly studies will be done. It's unclear why you gained forty pounds on Prempro. In my experience, women in their first year of hormone replacement therapy have a small weight gain. But one study showed that the average weight gain women who went on HRT experienced in the first year was two pounds, and women who did *not* go on HRT gained four pounds. Remember, metabolism is slowing at about 2 percent a year. I discuss what women can do about weight gain in chapter 6.

I'm still not sold on any kind of synthetic drug treatment for my menopause. What do you tell women who just say no to HRT or Raloxifene?

The need for a healthy lifestyle becomes even more important if you are not going to use HRT or Raloxifene. It's important that you don't smoke, eat a low-fat diet and increase your exercise. Medical checkups are important.

I have struggled with high blood pressure. My doctor would not prescribe estrogen pills because of that. What about Raloxifene?

I'm not sure why your doctor wouldn't prescribe estrogen. Years ago doctors wouldn't prescribe estrogen for high blood pressure. Now we feel that those women need it more than anyone else because they are at higher risk for stroke and heart disease. I would ask your doctor again why he or she feels you aren't a candidate for estrogen to make sure that this is the part of your medical history of concern.

I've read a lot about the "youthfulness" benefits of estrogen, especially for keeping a woman's skin and breasts looking young. Does Raloxifene have similar benefits? Or will I end up with bones of steel but be a wrinkled, sagging mess?

There're just no data yet. There is no evidence that it enhances better skin tone. If youthfulness is a main issue for you and that's why you're taking estrogen and doing well on it, then you are the kind of woman I tell, "Wait a year or two." If you're concerned about your skin and you're not taking estrogen, your question is probably, Will Raloxifene make it worse? There's certainly no evidence in the clinical trials that women complained about any aging of their skin. Raloxifene may not enhance the aging process, but I feel confident saying that it isn't going to accelerate it. I'm optimistic that it will give a lot of the benefits of estrogen, but the data are just not there yet.

FOUR

raloxifene and
how to take it

Recently a seventy-six-year-old woman came to see me for the first time. While taking her medical history, I asked her, "Are you on any medications?" She reached into her purse and pulled out this huge baggie. Inside she must have had ten bottles. She held them up to me, explaining how she was on this medicine for her blood pressure, and that medicine for her arthritis, and this one for gout. She had prescriptions for cholesterol lowering, for her ulcer, for her thyroid, and more, as well as some vitamins thrown in for good measure.

Later, when I discussed with her that there was a new medication that will build and preserve bone, lower cholesterol and reduce the risk of breast and uterine cancer, she interrupted me. "I like that! I get four things for one pill!" We both started to laugh.

If there was ever a pill that was "easy to swallow" Raloxifene is it. You can take Evista with or without food. You can take it morning, noon or night, at whatever time most meets your own schedule. Most people like to take medication at the same time each day because it becomes a habit that they can remember. But if you should miss a pill, there aren't big consequences. This drug has what's known as a long half-life—it will still be working for you a day after you've taken it.

Unlike Fosamax, the osteoporosis drug with the restrictions that you can't lie down or eat after you take it, Evista has no such requirements. You continue your normal activities.

As with any drug, it's important never to exceed the recommended dosage. More isn't better. Side effects are mentioned on the package insert, which you will want to read carefully. These include leg cramps and hot flashes. I don't want to minimize side effects—and you should report any to your doctor—but the incidence of these side effects in women taking Evista was very low, as discussed previously in chapter 2.

What are women who are currently taking Evista saying about it? Here's a sample of what I've been told by patients and other women since the release of the medication last January:

"It's much easier to be on, I feel, than the Tamoxifen I took for five and a half years following my lumpectomy. There was something about Tamoxifen that really felt like chemotherapy. Evista feels different, or milder, I'd say. I have gotten some mild hot flashes. But they are not at all like the ones I got on Tamoxifen, where I dripped so badly, my hair would get wet. No strange and scary discharges, either."

—K.C., *age fifty-eight*

"Prempro did something to my libido, I think. I was never in the mood for sex anymore and I couldn't think of any other reason why. I've been on Evista four months and I feel better already in that regard. I do feel a little warmer at night, and I don't know if that's what they mean by the fact that I might have some hot

flashes. I wouldn't call these flashes, but I never had them
anyway, so I wouldn't know. I'm happy with it, overall."

        —A.B., age fifty

"I feel great. I think I'm getting all the benefits of estrogen that
I'd heard about that I never got with Premarin and Provera
because I couldn't stand feeling bloated all of the time. And this
is one pill in a simple bottle. Less to remember. With all I have
on my mind these days, it's a definite bonus."

        —S.K., age fifty-four

"I had a hysterectomy at forty-two and was plunged right into
menopause. I took estrogen all of these years, but I got very
nervous when it was five years later, and I was still on the drug.
I heard the risks go up at that point. I started on Evista the week
after it came out. One thing makes me miss the estrogen—I'm
having vaginal dryness. But I just started using Estring and it's
helping. If I can get rid of that problem, I'll be home free."

        —B.A., age forty-eight

"My husband accuses me of being a hypochondriac. I read a lot.
I have a tendency to hear about the symptoms of a disease and
think I've got it. My doctor has told me more than once to take
my medical guides and throw them in the trash because they're
giving me more stress than relief. I'm just very in tune with my
body, and I feel subtle differences and worry about them when
other women might say, So what? I wasn't a great candidate for
estrogen. It was the breast cancer thing. I kept worrying about
my breasts and doing daily self-exams and then thinking
something could be so small I wouldn't feel it anyway. I never
refilled the prescription. For about three years I was on nothing
at all. That got me all worried because what was having no

estrogen going to mean for my bones and my heart? Evista made
sense for me. I wasn't going to take estrogen no matter what. I
don't know that I'm feeling much of anything since I started
taking it. I think that's a plus. I'm symptom-free."

—C.A., *age fifty-two*

As this book goes to press, women in the United States who started to take Evista right after its release will have been on it only eight months. Down the road, doctors will undoubtedly hear many more positive and negative reactions to Evista as we do with any drug we prescribe. These women's reactions are important. Scientists creating third- and fourth-generation SERMs, which I discuss in the last chapter of this book, will be listening closely.

For now, most of what I hear from women who are curious about Raloxifene are questions. Here are some of the most commonly asked questions about Evista and the answers:

Do I need to take Provera with Raloxifene?

Provera is necessary with traditional hormone replacement therapy for uterine protection. Estrogen causes proliferation (thickening) of the endometrial lining. If you take estrogen without progesterone to balance it over a long period of time, it can cause precancers and even cancers of the uterus. Progesterone is the drug that signals the uterus to slough off this lining, resulting in a "withdrawal bleed" not unlike a period. Therefore women who have a uterus have to take progesterone with estrogen to protect themselves.

Raloxifene does not cause the kind of proliferation and endometrial stimulation that estrogen does. Therefore you do not need to take progesterone with it. That's a relief for many women. Any form of progestin can cause breast tenderness and mood swings in many women, and it lowers the good cholesterol and raises the bad in all women.

I gained weight on HRT. What about Raloxifene?

In the clinical trial information that is available, there was no weight gain noted on Raloxifene.

I had a blood clot in my lung, and my doctor said I could not take estrogen. What about Raloxifene?

Unfortunately, as a Selective Estrogen Receptor Modulator, it appears that Raloxifene acts like estrogen on the venous side of the circulatory system. That is to say, there is a small increased risk of a blood clot in the veins that can travel to the lungs in women who take estrogen. The incidence is incredibly small, however, but women and their doctors need to be aware of it. This is important because if you have risk factors (previous blood clots; immobilization for a long period of time after an injury, fall or accident; or surgery that may diminish your mobility) you should not be on estrogens. Similarly you should not be on Raloxifene, either. It is not any *more* dangerous than estrogen, but not any less.

Will I still get my period on Raloxifene?

No. Raloxifene, unlike estrogen, does not stimulate the lining of the uterus. The reason that women on *sequential* hormone replacement therapy get their period is that estrogen stimulates the endometrial lining and then progesterone causes a withdrawal bleed, so that there will not be a buildup of endometrial tissue. This causes women to get their period. If women are on what is known as *continuous* combined HRT—where they take a small dose of progesterone all month long with the estrogen—about 60 to 70 percent of them will have no bleeding after three months. But the 30 to 40 percent who do have bleeding need to have some sort of biopsy or procedure, like a transvaginal sonogram, in order to prove that there is nothing abnormal going on in the uterus, causing the bleeding.

With Raloxifene there is no stimulation of the lining of the uterus and thus no bleeding. In the clinical trials there were no discontinuations in patients on the Raloxifene arm of the trials due to bleeding.

I feel pretty good. I am two years into menopause, I eat right and I exercise, and except for the fact that I don't menstruate, I can't tell the difference. Why should I take any drug?

Realize that there is a difference between taking medication for relief of menopausal symptoms (like hot flashes, insomnia or dry vagina) and the concept of taking a drug for health maintenance and prevention of disease.

Women who are postmenopausal will lose bone. This is because estrogen helps to inhibit the resorption of bone. Bone is a dynamic organ. For your entire life you are constantly laying down new bone cells and resorbing old bone cells. After menopause the rate of resorption is greater than the rate of new bone. So all women will lose bone. By age eighty, more than 50 percent of women will have osteoporosis as defined by the World Health Organization.

In addition, estrogen is known to lower cholesterol. Even if you have no problem with cholesterol, when you have estrogen on board, your cholesterol will be lower than it will be without estrogen.

Women who are premenopausal have a fraction of the heart attacks of men because of the presence of estrogen. After menopause, those who do not go on hormone replacement therapy catch up in terms of incidence of heart attacks relatively quickly. Thus there are tremendous benefits to having an estrogenic function for your entire life.

During menopause you no longer make estrogen because the ovaries have become quiescent. The concept of a drug that will give you the estrogenic function—in terms of preventing bone loss and lowering cholesterol, thus reducing heart disease—is very tempting. The reason, however, many, many women do not take estrogen, and the progesterone that is necessary with it, is because of fear of breast cancer. This may not be totally unfounded since recent evidence from the Nurses' Health Study indicates that women who take estrogen replacement therapy for more than ten years have a 30 to 40 percent increase in breast cancer. In addition, many women have breast tenderness and a feeling of bloating from HRT. And finally, many women on HRT have cyclical or unexplained uterine bleeding, which is a nuisance and can lead to the need for further medical interventions to prove that there isn't any serious pathology inside the uterus.

Thus many women don't want to take any kind of medication. However the concept of a drug that can give you many of the benefits that estrogen normally confers without the risks, and that reduces the risk of breast cancer at the same time, is a very exciting concept for health maintenance.

I am worried about osteoporosis, but I would rather take some natural forms of hormones. Isn't Raloxifene synthetic?

Raloxifene is a synthetic Selective Estrogen Receptor Modulator. The change of the configuration of the molecules slightly in the laboratory is what enables it to be recognized as estrogen in tissues where you want estrogen and recognized as an estrogen blocker in tissues where you don't want estrogen. So, yes, it is synthetic. But I believe this is an example of better living through chemistry. If I can create a better chemical molecule, the fact that something is made in the laboratory doesn't disturb me. Natural is not the same as being risk-free. If you take natural forms of hormones, they are still metabolized by your liver. Plus you don't know the potency or the effective dose that you're getting and its effect on your breasts and your uterus.

In your question you said that you are worried about osteoporosis. Women with such concerns should be doing weight-bearing exercise and taking calcium and vitamin D regularly. But certainly a preventive agent like Raloxifene would offer some tremendous potential advantages.

I had breast cancer nine years ago. I am on Fosamax. Can I take Raloxifene with it/instead of it?

Most women who have had breast cancer in the past should not and will not want to take traditional hormone replacement therapy. Many of these women are losing bone. Some are taking Fosamax, either for prevention of osteoporosis or for treatment of known osteoporosis.

If you are on Fosamax for known osteoporosis, then you should continue with it. There are no studies that indicate that adding Raloxifene to it will be more beneficial for your bone density.

However, the Fosamax that you are on will do nothing to reduce your cholesterol, possibly prevent heart disease and prevent new-onset breast cancer in your contralateral breast.

Many women in your situation elect to take Raloxifene either with or instead of Fosamax, depending on their bone density. Although I recognize that there are currently no studies that indicate that it will be effective for you to take this combination, I personally believe there is no harm in combining Fosamax with Raloxifene or estrogen, for that matter. They are all antiresorptives. Although using multiple antiresorptives may improve bone mineral density, there are as yet no data to indicate that it will reduce fractures.

As your doctor, it would be important for me to know what your bone mineral density is before advising you. If you are on Fosamax for prevention of osteoporosis, then you certainly could take Raloxifene instead of Fosamax because Raloxifene will prevent bone loss and osteoporosis as well as lower cholesterol and act as potent antiestrogen for your other breast.

I had breast cancer four years ago, and I am on Tamoxifen. I had an abnormal transvaginal ultrasound eighteen months ago but a D&C showed nothing. Is Raloxifene for me?

Realize that Tamoxifen is the most widely prescribed antineoplastic drug worldwide. It will save lives, it will prolong lives, it will prolong disease-free intervals in women with breast cancer. It does, however, form some uterine cancers in women.

My expertise initially was in transvaginal ultrasound. I can assure you that many, many more women get an abnormal *picture* on transvaginal ultrasound than those who in fact have any true uterine abnormality. There is a difference between having an abnormal ultrasound picture and having a disease process in the uterus. In work that I have done, as many as 25 percent of women will have a funny-looking ultrasound with nothing wrong. In addition, upwards of 40 percent of women will develop nonmalignant changes of the uterus on Tamoxifen.

But I realize this is a very emotional issue. You have already had one malignancy. Now you are told you have an abnormality in the uterus while you are on a drug that is known to increase your risk of uterine cancer. Having a D&C, even if it showed nothing, is a very traumatic thing to go through. I have had patients who have said to me that even though the D&C showed benign findings, they refuse to stay on Tamoxifen.

If that is the case, I would rather see you go on Raloxifene than be on nothing at all, because I believe that Raloxifene will be beneficial. Studies are being done, and I firmly believe that within five years we will be using Raloxifene or more likely third-generation SERMs as a treatment for women with breast cancer the way we use Tamoxifen now. But I cannot advise you in good faith to stop a proven drug to go on one that hasn't been proven yet. But, if because of the emotional issues that I've just outlined, you are planning to stop Tamoxifen of your own volition, I would rather see you be on Raloxifene than on nothing at all.

I have been on Prempro for three years, but my mom had breast cancer at age fifty-four. If I switch to Raloxifene, will I get hot flashes? If so, what can I do?

I hear this from many, many of my patients. Women who are on hormone replacement therapy for its numerous benefits often go on it reluctantly because of a strong family history of breast cancer. Many women like yourself want to switch to Raloxifene.

There are not abundant data on how great the incidence of hot flashes is to be expected in someone on HRT who switches to Raloxifene. In women who were given Raloxifene who were on no other drugs prior to treatment, the incidence of hot flashes was about 25 percent, but the flashes tended to be mild and not last more than six months. It is uncertain what the incidence would be in a group containing women like yourself.

Current recommendations are to come off of Prempro for four weeks to let it wash out of your system, and then make the transition to Raloxifene. The more gradual the change from estrogen to Raloxifene, the less likely you will be to have hot flashes. Regardless, it appears that the hot flashes will be mild in severity and, it is hoped, not long-lived.

What if you do have uncomfortable, persistent hot flashes? Can you take a small dose of estrogen with the Raloxifene to prevent the hot flashes or treat them without undoing the protective effect on the breast? Once again, there are no firm data on this. But it appears that the breast protective issue is dose related. A full dose of Raloxifene is 60 milligrams, but it is unclear how much estrogen is necessary to undue the breast protection issue. From a breast point of view, a half dose of estrogen (0.3 mg) might not absolutely equal one half of a 60-mg dose of Raloxifene. Furthermore mixing estrogen and Raloxifene might be additive or pose an even greater risk in terms of deep-vein thrombosis.

I am on medication for high blood pressure. Can I take Raloxifene with it?

There is no problem from a drug/drug interaction perspective. Furthermore, because of your high blood pressure you are at increased risk for heart disease. Raloxifene has clearly been shown to lower cholesterol and other surrogate markers for cardiovascular disease. There are currently ongoing studies to see and prove definitively if Raloxifene can in fact reduce heart disease directly and not just through surrogate markers.

A generation ago, women with high blood pressure were told not to take estrogen because there was some fear that it could increase their risks. Now women with high blood pressure are some of the first patients doctors suggest go on HRT for protection against cardiac disease.

I have heard that the other osteoporosis drug, Fosamax, can cause upset stomach. I have a sensitive stomach. Is Raloxifene a problem?

Raloxifene does not cause any gastrointestinal distress. It can be taken on a full stomach or an empty stomach. It is well absorbed. It can be taken at night or in the morning. There are no restrictions regarding being able to lie down after you take it. It has a relatively long half-life, so that if you forget one day it is not a problem.

I am seventy-seven years old. I never took hormones. When I went through my changes they said, "Hormones cause cancer." My bone density test is slightly low, but the doctor said I don't have osteoporosis. Is it too late to start Raloxifene?

No, not at all. Raloxifene is not yet approved as a treatment for osteoporosis. But for someone like you who doesn't yet have osteoporosis, Raloxifene is an excellent choice for *preservation* of bone. In addition, Raloxifene can still give you the benefit of lowering your lipids and not stimulating your breasts and in fact probably reducing your risk of breast cancer, a disease whose incidence goes up and up as you get older. In addition, one of the problems for people in your age group with traditional HRT is that it is very difficult to take someone who has not had a period in twenty-six years and expect her to get any degree of vaginal bleeding.

So no one is ever too old to start Raloxifene. The fact that it doesn't cause uterine bleeding should make it much easier to tolerate, and if you don't already have osteoporosis, it will be an excellent way to prevent its development.

I am forty-seven years old. My mom and both her sisters had breast cancer in their fifties. Can I start Raloxifene now even though my periods are still regular?

No, unfortunately not. Raloxifene is simply for women who are *postmenopausal*. It is not approved and it is not a good idea to give it to women who are still cycling. Its exact effects in women who are still cycling are unclear, although Tamoxifen given to such women can cause an increase in endometriosis and a growth in fibroids.

The national average of menopause is 51.4. Many women in my practice who are your age and who have large fibroid uteri, have been told that they need hysterectomies. They have opted for supracervical hysterectomies (where the cervix is left intact) and preservation of their ovaries in order to maintain ovarian function, in your case for another 4.4 years on average.

Recently a woman just like you who needed a supracervical hysterectomy for her fibroids said to me, "While you're in there please take my ovaries out so that I can go on Raloxifene. I want to protect my breasts from cancer." She no longer wanted ovarian function because she knew if her ovaries were removed, then she would not have to wait until natural menopause to go on Raloxifene and get the breast protective effect.

This may seem radical to some women, but realize that there are women whose history of breast cancer is as great as yours and who have already had prophylactic double mastectomies in order to try to prevent breast cancer. The concept of placing two extra clamps to take the ovaries out "if you are already in there" for a diseased uterus, so that you can go on a breast cancer–protective agent is, maybe, a lot more appealing than preventive mastectomies, which many women have, in fact, undergone.

I tend to have oily skin. Birth control pills gave me acne. What will Raloxifene do?

Oily skin and development of acne were not reported as results of Raloxifene in the clinical trials. It appears from the anecdotal information currently available that taking Raloxifene does not result in increased oily skin or acne.

My dad had Alzheimer's. Is Raloxifene as good as estrogen for my brain?

Once again, this has not been well studied, and we hope that data will be forthcoming soon. Realize that any FDA decision to approve a drug is based upon proof that it is efficacious and safe. The drug claims to prevent osteoporosis, to lower lipids and to be safe to the breast and the uterus. I have given you my interpretation of data that have been presented in the public forum. Alzheimer's is a tragic disease. Plenty of data suggest that estrogen may prevent

Alzheimer's. The data for this are not nearly as strong, or what we call "hard," as the data for estrogen preserving bone, lowering lipids, or even increasing the risk for breast cancer. Raloxifene appears to be absorbed in the gray matter of the brain the same way estrogen is. Based on limited data, it is my opinion and hope that when more data are in fact available, whatever it is that estrogen does for the brain, Raloxifene will do as well.

Lately I have noticed my hair seems to be falling out. How will Raloxifene affect my hair?

There appeared to be no increased complaints of hair loss in any of the Raloxifene groups compared to those on the placebo. If Raloxifene caused hair changes, one would expect that it would have been a commonly reported side effect of women in the clinical trials.

I stopped Premarin because my breasts were killing me. Will Raloxifene have the same effect?

No. It absolutely should not. Almost all breast tenderness that women experience when they take estrogen is related to the stimulatory effect of estrogen on breast and breast ductual tissue. Raloxifene is a potent antiestrogen in breasts. From a scientific theoretical point of view, one would not expect to see any breast tenderness. Furthermore, in the clinical trials this was almost never reported as a side effect in any of the Raloxifene groups, whereas those trials that involved estrogen did report significant rates of breast tenderness.

I am three years postmenopausal. Sex is uncomfortable because I am so dry. Will Raloxifene help?

Raloxifene is not a treatment for vaginal dryness. Since Raloxifene doesn't seem to treat hot flashes either, there is concern as to whether Raloxifene might exacerbate vaginal dryness. In the clinical trials, however, there appeared to be no increase whatsoever in vaginal dryness associated with Raloxifene. Women in the clinical trials, regardless of which group they were in, were allowed to use vaginal estrogen cream if they felt they were dry vaginally. The incidence of use of vaginal estrogen cream in the Raloxifene and placebo groups was virtually identical.

I am on Premarin and Provera. I have decided to switch to Raloxifene. Can I just start Evista right away?

If you are on sequential HRT, you are cycling, and the cycle finishes when you finish the progesterone (in your case, Provera). So, don't just quit somewhere in the middle and start Raloxifene. Finish the progesterone, after which you'll get your withdrawal bleed, and then wait four weeks from the last pill to let the drugs wash out of your body. Then you can start Raloxifene.

Raloxifene sounds like a great product. Why couldn't men take it?

That was one of the first questions that I asked. Certainly men get osteoporosis, although not nearly as much as women. Men can certainly benefit from a reduction in cholesterol and heart disease. It would depend on the effect of Raloxifene on the prostate gland. It doesn't cause any breast stimulation as would happen if men took estrogen. If a man took estrogen, he would tend to develop gynecomastia (enlargement of the breasts).

There are absolutely no data on the use of Raloxifene in men. However, I am hopeful that new SERMs will be developed that will be tested and used in men. And I look forward to perhaps some day taking a third-generation SERM for health maintenance as I approach my sunset years.

FIVE

boosting the benefits

Whether or not you decide to take Raloxifene, you have options for dealing with menopausal symptoms, ones that Raloxifene may or may not affect. This chapter will give you the best remedies for the health challenges that women who reach menopause face.

WHAT TO DO ABOUT HOT FLASHES AND NIGHT SWEATS

Hot flashes are definite signs that your supply of estrogen has dwindled. The hypothalamus, the heat-regulating center in the brain, interprets low estrogen levels as a drop in body temperature. It responds by triggering mechanisms to warm you up. Blood rushes to the skin. You flush. The sensation can quickly travel through your whole body. While sometimes very uncomfortable, even bad flashes are not medically dangerous to you.

Night sweats are hot flashes that happen when you're sleeping. You wake up sweating, sometimes your heart is beating fast, and you may have an overall sense of disorientation. Don't be surprised if your side of the bed feels absolutely wet. This doesn't mean anything dangerous has happened.

1. Try vitamins. Vitamin C (time released, 2,000 mg per day), vitamin E (400 international units in dry form) and vitamin B complex are all helpful in reducing hot flashes. If you are already taking multivitamins, check how much you are already adding to your system and do the math before you add more, because higher levels aren't going to help.

2. Ask your doctor about other medications for hot flashes. For some women, hot flashes aren't so terrible. But I've known patients who were having so many of them a day that they were completely disruptive to their lives.

Estrogen is still the best medical science has to offer in treating hot flashes. Beyond that, your doctor may mention Megestrol or Bellergal. Megestrol acetate is a synthetic female hormone doctors have prescribed for years to treat breast and endometrial cancer. Some doctors do prescribe Megestrol for women who can't take HRT—usually women with breast cancer. In a study published in *The New England Journal of Medicine*, researchers at the Mayo Clinic found that the drug reduced the frequency and severity of hot flashes 85 percent of the time. However, side effects reported include abnormal menstrual bleeding.

Bellergal is a drug that has been proven effective at reducing hot flashes. It also reduces nervousness, dizziness, irritability and palpitations. However, it contains Phenobarbital, something that can be habit-forming. It also isn't recommended for women with high blood pressure, heart disease or kidney or liver problems.

Clonidine, which is also available in a patch, is a medication for high blood pressure which some women find helpful. However, the side effects include dry mouth, dizziness and insomnia.

3. Avoid red wine, chocolate, caffeine, white sugar and alcohol. These are well-known hot-flash triggers for many women. Go without them for two weeks, and see how you feel.

4. Sleep in a cool room. If you're already in a thermostat war with your partner, point out that while a person can always cover up in extra blankets to get warmer in a cold room, a woman going through a phase of hot flashes can do nothing to ease those waves of warmth in a hot room with no ventilation. A cooperative mate should understand why the thermostat should be turned down during this time-limited period. You may need separate blankets you can kick off without disturbing another person's sleep. Forget the top sheet. Regardless of the thread count, it usually doesn't breathe and you can wake up feeling like you're wrapped in plastic in a pool of sweat.

5. Dress in layers so that you can peel clothes off or put them back on as the need arises. Go for cotton, which absorbs moisture and allows heat to escape. Choose summer-weight nylons, and stock up on them for the winter.

6. Buy a personal fan. Portable desk fans, available for about ten dollars at drugstores, are becoming high tech. Some fans even mist you with cool water. You can put them in the freezer at night and have a cool spray that lasts hours. You'll hardly be alone in using them. An eighth-grade teacher told me this story: "The air-conditioning went on the blink during a terribly hot day in September, and the entire class was drenched and cranky by the end of the day. The next morning, more than fifteen kids walked in with these little battery-operated portable fans in all shapes and sizes. Where did they borrow them from? Their mothers!"

Freeze those facial napkins that come in little packets and carry them with you. Use them to cool your pulse points (your wrists, your neck). This often works better than gliding them across your face.

7. Don't stop exercising. You might think, Who needs to flush and sweat any more than this? But exercise can also raise the level of activity of endorphins in the body—those natural mood lifters that relax and comfort—which may alleviate hot flashes.

8. Know your own triggers. If stress is one, then this is not the time to sign up to give a speech at the community college, redo your kitchen or host your family reunion. This symptom will pass, so if you can get out of a stressful event now, do it.

9. Consider Progestin alone. It won't be as effective as estrogen and progestins together, but it helps many women. Depo-Provera, an injectable form of progestin, has been found to relieve hot flashes in 89.5 percent of women. Side effects such as headaches or abnormal bleeding are pretty common, however.

SOOTHING VAGINAL DRYNESS

Sometimes a strange new dryness is the first symptom women get that says: This is truly it—menopause. You don't feel dry because you aren't interested in having sex; you notice a dryness all the time that you can feel, sometimes even just walking.

Infection, irritation and discomfort can come from this sudden dryness. To ward them off, try the following:

- Wear cotton underwear and cotton-crotch nylons. They allow more air to circulate.

- Use KY jelly, Astroglide (a favorite among many of my patients) or Replens, as often as you have to. They can make you feel more comfortable, even when sexual activity isn't the primary motivation.

- Vitamin E cream and/or Vitamin E 100-600IU can be helpful for more lubrication. Omega-3 fatty acids (fish oils) are a remedy that some women claim helps retain all-over hydration.

- Exercise increases circulation to the pelvic area. So does regular sex. Don't avoid sex and think you'll come back to it later. The vaginal wall stays healthier in women who remain sexually active. Sexual arousal produces some natural lubrication, and sexual activity increases blood flow to the area, which helps keep the vaginal tissues supple.

- Antihistamines, which dry your running nose, can dry your whole body, including your vagina, so be aware of this if you use them regularly. Deodorant soaps, douches and hygiene sprays can also be drying.

- Drink enough water to keep your body hydrated. Six glasses a day is a minimum! This is healthy for every part of your body.

GETTING YOUR CHOLESTEROL DOWN

Postmenopausal women are more vulnerable to heart disease because estrogen affects blood cholesterol levels. Total cholesterol levels of postmenopausal women are about 25mg/dl (that's milligrams per deciliter—yes, you're in the metric system here) higher than in women who have not reached menopause.

It's important to know your numbers. When you have your

cholesterol tested, you should get a score for total cholesterol, HDL (high-density lipoprotein), LDL (low-density lipoprotein) and triglycerides. This is what you need to know.

Total cholesterol: If your reading is about 200 mg/dl, you're in the normal range. More than 240 is considered high. Heart attacks are very uncommon in people who have cholesterol levels of 150 or lower, but that number may be very difficult to achieve.

HDL: Normal is 35 mg/dl and above. You don't want to have less than 35, because too little HDL can allow plaque to accumulate in your arteries. If your score is higher than 60 mg/dl, you're doing great. If your HDL is too low, try getting more aerobic exercise—at least thirty minutes three or four times a week.

LDL: Below 130 mg/dl is considered good. More than 160 is considered too high for your health. If your LDL is too high, cut saturated fat in your diet to about 10 percent of your total calories. This means avoiding red meat and high-fat dairy products, such as many cheeses.

Triglycerides: There's a wider acceptable range here. If you're anywhere between 85 mg/dl to 200 mg/dl, you're in a normal, healthy range. Past 400, and you need to look at ways to lower it.

A healthy goal would be to get your triglyceride level under 100 mg/dl. If it isn't there now, cut down on refined flours and sugars. Make your diet heavy in whole grains, fruits and vegetables.

Add as much garlic and soy products as you can. The key here is making regular changes in your diet. A Caesar salad laden with garlic once a week isn't going to do it. Walking the stairs instead of taking the elevator when the thought crosses your mind is great for the moment, but not the kind of steady exercise that will make a difference.

You've tried making changes in your diet, and exercising, but it still isn't helping? There are some supplements that may help. Niacin, or vitamin B3, may help to reduce LDL cholesterol and

Calcium supplements are another way to get your daily intake up where it needs to be. Tums, an over-the-counter antacid, for example, is 100 percent calcium carbonate with only a little added flavoring. Chewing four a day will do the trick, and it will be better absorbed if you take it four times a day rather than all at once. Stay away from antacids that also contain aluminum, because these actually get in the way of the intestine's ability to absorb calcium from food. Diets high in protein and very high in certain types of fiber, such as wheat bran, can also inhibit calcium absorption. So can a high intake of alcohol and salt.

One note of caution: Since these supplements are so easy to chew and swallow, don't decide that the more the better. Very high calcium levels can cause constipation and may interfere with the body's absorption of iron and zinc. Normal calcium metabolism requires adequate vitamin D. Standard supplementation is 400 IU per day.

Calcium content of selected foods:

1 cup yogurt	415 mg
3 oz. Parmesan cheese	335 mg
1 cup juice fortified with calcium	300 mg
1 cup milk	300 mg
1 oz. Cheddar cheese	205 mg
1 oz. Swiss cheese	270 mg
1 cup ice cream	175 mg
1 egg	55 mg
4 oz. tofu	155 mg
3 oz. canned salmon	210 mg

Many women reach menopause and battle with weight gain. It's a well-researched fact that a woman's metabolism slows down 2 percent a year in middle age. "These days I *look* at food and gain weight," one patient told me. She's not far off. Do the math, and it's clear why women who don't eat any more or exercise any less than they did at forty-five may be ten pounds heavier at fifty-five.

"I have been walking half an hour a day for the last five years," a patient told me, distressed that it no longer did much for her weight. She didn't love hearing this, but I had to tell her the truth: "At your age you may have to do an hour a day, and that's just to keep what you have."

Added to this easy-gain, hard-loss reality is the fact that a woman's weight is going to shift to different places as she grows older, and the shift is more obvious in thinner women. "I spent my twenties and thirties complaining about the cellulite in my thighs. It dawned on me the other day that my thighs haven't looked this good in years. But I have this little growing pot belly. My old strategy—a week of low-calorie microwave lunches, no chips or snacks, and a half an hour walk a day, and there go five pounds—just didn't work. In fact, I gained two pounds. I used to feel pride that I didn't even know how to do crunches because my stomach was flat as a board. Now I'm doing a hundred fifty crunches a day; it's slow going and it feels like my breasts are getting fat." It isn't her imagination. Nature distributed your fat where it determined it was needed most for procreation. When estrogen production stops, the pear-shaped woman often turns into the apple shaped woman, much to her chagrin.

You can't work against what nature decided is the best distribution of fat for continuing the species by wishing it was different.

And you are going to have to deal with the real ramifications of that slower metabolism, which often means that when you're fifty-five you are ten pounds heavier than you were at forty-five and you've done absolutely nothing differently.

As a doctor, I see daily how excessive weight takes its toll on both physical and mental health. I also know that women who have reached their fifties and still struggle with weight gain have tried just about everything under the sun, and they need an entirely new approach. After all, doing the same thing over and over again and expecting a different result is a setup for failure.

Should you diet at all? In the past decade we've seen an anti-dieting movement. It has its roots in studies of so-called yo-yo dieting, in which people actually got fatter each time they went off a diet than they were when they started. Still, to say never diet is as extreme as saying go on a juice fast for the next month. The healthiest way to lose weight is to reduce your calories and increase your exercise. In my experience, many people need to at least start off with some type of diet plan because they need some parameters. Diets aren't merely restrictions but models for how to eat in a manner that is balanced, contains healthy variety and includes moderation. The secret to keeping the weight off is to make this a lifestyle change rather than a "diet."

What about low-fat diets? The warnings against dietary fat stem from cholesterol concerns. Carbohydrates are the easiest to convert into body fat. For many people, low fat has become high carbohydrate.

It is proteins that are the hardest of all to be converted to fat. However, the overfed body will convert them. At the end of the day, it's calories in and calories out. Whether you eat 800 calories of cheesecake or 800 calories of carrot sticks, you still get 800 calories. I've seen women gain weight on a low-fat diet, also because they are loading themselves up with low-fat cookies and low-fat chips.

Severe salt restriction is one of the best things a woman can do for her body. Our diets are much too high in sodium. The sodium contained in most foods that you buy in a prepared fashion or in restaurants is sufficient to cause water retention. Water retention in different organ systems gives multiple symptoms. One is weight gain. Another is mood swings and headache. In the breast it causes breast tenderness. Generally it can cause bloating and cramps.

If you have a significant amount of weight to lose, I recommend that you do it in stages. Lose part of the weight you need to lose and stay there. Stay there, if need be, for a whole year. Prove to yourself that you won't gain it back. Then work on losing the next part. It can be much more motivating to make your goal losing five pounds at a time. First of all, it's a goal most people can reach. Setting out to lose thirty pounds can be overwhelming.

Elisabeth Halfpapp, vice president of the Lotte Berk Method, with exercise studios in New York City, the Hamptons and Greenwich and New Canaan, Connecticut, has this advice for women past menopause who are looking to lose weight: "First get muscle. Muscle needs more calories just to function anatomically. Once you increase your muscle density, your metabolic rate increases and in turn you start to burn calories more efficiently. When a woman comes to me and says, I want to lose weight, I want to stop smoking, I want to stop drinking, I want to go on a diet, I tell her one step at a time. Start by building muscle. It's amazing how when women do this, things just fall into place."

Most women have lost considerable muscle mass by the time they reach their fifties. Beginning in your thirties, a combination of hormonal changes and a lower activity level cause women to lose lean muscle mass each year, which slows the metabolic rate so that food is burned less efficiently. Even if you do exercise, less muscle mass means you burn fewer calories.

The Lotte Berk Method is a sports-training, strengthening program based on the balance of strengthening and stretching exercises that can help women counteract this. The exercises are taken from the disciplines of ballet, modern dance, yoga and orthopedic back exercises. The goal is to tone muscles, stretch muscles and redistribute weight. It uses your own body—not weights or machines—with an emphasis on correct alignment and posture.

I have taken Lotte Berk Method classes, and in my opinion the method is one of the best programs not only for building muscle but also for improving flexibility. Flexibility is going to be to the year 2000 what aerobics was to the eighties, as we age and wonder, "Am I going to be able to get out of the backseat of a car a decade from now? Or pick up my grandchild in my arms?"

In addition to improving flexibility, the method redistributes weight and helps women lose inches in the right places. Says Elisabeth, who has been teaching the method for more than a decade: "Many women in their fifties and sixties have said to me, "My body isn't going to change at this point. This is just the way it is." It's not true. If they do the right exercise and they really are consistent with it, the changes happen."

Elisabeth believes that the right kind of exercise is this combination of stretching and strengthening, especially once a woman reaches menopause. "I really believe they should not run or jog. I think it puts a lot of strain on the female organs. It ages you, it breaks down the elasticity of your skin. It makes you look stressed. I used to run ten miles every other day when I was in my twenties. I remember the last time I ran. I looked in the mirror afterwards and I looked so strained, so worn. The stress in my face made me look twenty years older. With these exercises, women leave with a relaxed, calm energy."

But do they lose weight? "Definitely. And they lose inches. I have seen women literally transform their bodies. Every day it amazes me the changes I see happen, not just physically and aesthetically but orthopedically. I remember one woman who came in with the worst back condition, who'd had surgeries, and who couldn't do much of anything where her back wouldn't be in pain. She was gaining weight, feeling horrible about herself. She was able to do a lot of the work at the studio, in spite of her back condition. Six weeks later it was like her body was transformed, it was like a shell had been shed from her body. She gained confidence from being able to reshape her body in a safe way. I was working with a woman in her fifties several years ago, who came in almost ready to develop a dowager's hump. Her posture today is like a ballet dancer's. Do these exercises for an hour three times a week and in six weeks you will definitely see changes in your body."

The exercises are fully described in the book *The Lotte Berk Method*, by Lydia Bach, and is available by calling the studio. Women with back problems will find exercises geared to toning weakened stomach muscles, which relieves pressure on the back. The method even includes exercises to improve sexual agility, comfort and confidence.

GETTING THE SLEEP YOU NEED

When women reach menopause, they often don't sleep as well as they once did because of the estrogen deficiency. Two very common problems are having trouble falling asleep and waking in the middle of the night and being unable to fall back to sleep sometimes for an hour or two.

It's true that women who take estrogen often report that they sleep better. We have no research yet on what will happen to women on Raloxifene in terms of their sleep. There are, however, some things women can do to improve their chances of getting a good night's rest.

1. Wake up at the same time every day. If that doesn't help, wake up half an hour earlier. This is easier said than done. You've tossed and turned, perhaps because of night sweats or tension and ended up watching the four-o'-clock movie. Just as the alarm goes off, you finally feel sleepy. Forget thinking that you need those eight hours and deciding to crawl back in bed. You will do more damage to your body clock and eventual body well-being by over-sleeping. For many women, the key to not being able to fall asleep is getting up even earlier. Force yourself to keep a regular schedule, and you'll reap the benefits of deeper sleep.

2. Beware of hidden caffeine. Chocolate is one source of caffeine that can keep you awake. I know a woman who had a serious thing for M&M's. She kept the candy dish in her den full of them. They were for guests, she said, but she used to get up in the middle of the night to go to the bathroom, and grab a handful on the way and another handful on the way back. She was surprised to learn it was the caffeine, not guilt over the little nighttime chocolate binges, that gave her trouble getting back to sleep.

Excedrin before bedtime keeps some women up for hours. And read the ingredients of cold medicines. The over-the-counter-lose-weight-quick pills of too many names and varieties to list are also often full of caffeine.

3. Make your largest meal lunch. Why add major digestion to your nighttime list of things your body needs to do to finally settle down and relax enough to sleep. The full stomach that makes you nod off in front of the TV at seven at night has a habit of waking you up just when you gather yourself up off the couch and head for bed.

4. Use your bed for sleep, and nothing else. Don't eat in bed. Don't take your laptop into bed to do work. Don't read memos in bed or write letters or otherwise make your bed a surrogate office. Don't make your bed the place where your children bounce in and tell you how the science fair project due tomorrow and the poster you worked on for hours got left on the bus. Don't fight with your partner in bed. Don't seethe in bed, and pretend to be asleep. Don't read in bed, either, unless you are the type of reader who reads at night to make your eyes tired, and this is a nightly ritual you can count on to make you feel tired. Consider moving the TV out of the bedroom. When you can't sleep, get out of bed and go to another room and sit there for as long as it takes for you to really want to go back to bed, to sleep. The key is to get mental stimulation out of your bed and into other rooms of your house, so that you come to see the bed as a place of peace and rest. It may take about twenty-one days to do this—the time period scientists suggest it takes to form a new habit.

5. Fill your bedroom with soothing sound. There are devices called "Sound Soothers" that can fill your room with white noise, or restful sounds of nature such as waves and waterfalls. These sounds help many people drift off to sleep and mask unwanted noises throughout the night. You plug them in, and dial the sound you prefer. They can play for either half an hour or all night, depending on your setting. You may find you achieve a deeper sleep than you've had in months. And, if you place the device close to your pillow, you can drown out your snoring partner.

6. When you're awake, be fully awake. Realize that how you feel in your waking state has much to do with how you fare in your sleeping state. In his book *Restful Sleep*, Deepak Chopra wrote: "The solution to all sleep problems lies in making the period of daily activity truly dynamic and satisfying. In other words, when you're awake, be fully awake and alive." To Chopra, this is the fundamental answer to insomnia and the solution for many of the apparent problems of life as well. When you've learned to experience a pure wakefulness, liveliness and dynamism, good sleep will come naturally.

7. Try natural remedies. Vitamin C, vitamin B complex, and vitamin E work for some women. Others swear by melatonin. Don't forget the old standbys—a glass of warm milk or a hot bath before bed.

8. If insomnia is a serious problem, see your doctor. Definitely discuss your sleep problem with your gynecologist. If you've done that, and your problem persists, ask yourself if your insomnia is disrupting your life enough to consider seeing a doctor who is a sleep specialist. With thousands of Americans who only need to turn a light out to undergo six hours of major agitation, these appointments aren't that easy to get.

What's it like to go to a "sleep clinic"? A patient told me this: "I saw the specialist after a three-month bout of waking at three and not being able to fall back to sleep. She wanted to know everything about my patterns, the exact nature of my sleep. It was funny, but she wasn't the least bit interested in my theories about why this was happening, or about my mother's chronic insomnia. When I asked her why, she said what was significant wasn't *why* I wasn't sleeping but how to quickly restore natural rhythms of sleep. The prescription I was given was for trazodone. She said it wasn't habit-forming, wouldn't hang me over or make me dependent. And it *did* work for me. After three weeks of decent sleep, I stopped taking it, and I was able to sleep naturally. Now I only take it occasionally."

WHAT TO DO ABOUT DEPRESSION

Researchers contend that there is no direct link between depression and menopause. While I do not generally see many patients whose symptoms fit the clinical definition of depression, there are quite a few who complain of sudden tears at inopportune times, irritability and a lingering feeling of emptiness or sadness. Naturally one may have very real, very understandable feelings about growing older, about losing fertility, about having annoying symptoms. Add to that the fact that occasional blue moods are a part of life.

In my experience, bouts of depressed feelings tend to be at their worst during the transition into menopause. In fact, once a woman finally reaches menopause and gets beyond the symptoms, either through medication or other management, she often reports a new sense of well-being, not unlike a "second wind." The North American Menopause Society (NAMS) released the results of a 1997 survey conducted by the Gallup Organization, which found after interviewing a sample of women ages forty-five to sixty that 52 percent of them saw menopause as the beginning of a new and fulfilling state of life.

What if it's not going that well for you? First, rule out clinical depression, since 10 million Americans suffer from it, and the depression rate in the United States is nearly twice as high for women as it is for men.

When psychiatrists diagnose depression in a patient, they look for the following features, based on *The Diagnostic and Statistical Manual of Mental Disorders*, the "bible" of the field: depressed, hopeless mood; loss of pleasure and interest in almost all activities; significant weight loss or weight gain; sleeping too much or not being able to fall asleep; loss of energy; problems concentrating or making decisions; thoughts of death or suicide; agitation; or loss of affect. A patient must have at least five of these criteria, and have been experiencing them for at least two weeks.

One may look at that list and conclude, "That's me!" and yet not truly be suffering from depression. It's the degree of these symptoms, and the fact that they so often occur together without anything to provoke them that makes the difference. A doctor who specializes in depression can make a better diagnosis than the person suffering from it can. And a doctor who sees clinical depression every day can separate the characteristics of a bad case of the blues from a depression and often give you calming reassurance.

When I was in medical school I was taught that a key indication that a patient is depressed is that you begin to feel depressed when you are with him or her! Of course I don't go around diagnosing depression in everyone who depresses me, but don't overlook it if people close to you begin to ask you what's wrong, or tell you that you don't seem to be yourself. Many depressions are characterized by an absence of feeling rather than an overwhelming sadness. It's like a shutting down of the self because there are no more resources to battle the problems or feelings. Since the person doesn't feel much of anything, the thought that this is depression doesn't always naturally occur. Her more compelling thoughts are, "Who cares? Why bother? I'm tired—leave me alone."

See your doctor if you're concerned about depression. Today's medical treatments for depression have demonstrated unparalleled success when compared to what was available in our youth. They include a combination of psychotherapy and drug treatment. Paxil, Prozac, Zoloft and Serzone are common antidepressant medications known as "serotonin reuptake inhibitors." The brain has a natural level of certain neurotransmitters, one of which is serotonin. The brain breaks down serotonin as a natural process. There is a theory that in some people the brain breaks down the serotonin too quickly, causing a depressed feeling. There have been studies on lab animals that show some indication that a drop in estrogen may cause a corresponding drop in serotonin, although much more research needs to be done before we can conclude that this is also true in humans. Antidepressants balance the supply of serotonin, slowing its breakdown. They don't supply extra serotonin, but help you keep what you have a little longer. Thousands of people report relief, without a "drugged" feeling or abnormal feelings of euphoria. These drugs are not addictive and contain fewer side effects than previous medications for depression. They also work more quickly. And when they do work, they don't give you a feeling of euphoria. Chances are you won't feel unlike yourself, but more like your real self.

You're leery of medication? There is also growing talk among experts in the field of mood disorders about the herbal remedy known as St. John's Wort. You've likely heard about this herbal depression antidote that is popular in Germany. If you frequent health food stores, you have probably seen signs, "We Have St. John's Wort" everywhere. Like Paxil or Prozac, it appears to work by acting on the serotonin receptors. There have been studies that show that it's as effective as pharmaceutical antidepressants with moderate depression, especially when the major symptom is low energy. It's available at health food stores and is widely used throughout Europe. One capsule is taken three times a day. The study of this herb is ongoing, and it's certainly worth discussing with your doctor. If you are taking Prozac, Paxil or something else, definitely talk with your doctor before you switch to St. John's Wort.

If you are diagnosed with depression, and feel bad because you cannot shake off the blues by yourself, experts Harold H. Bloomfield, M.D., and Peter McWilliams, authors of *How to Heal Depression,* offer these empathic words in their highly acclaimed book: "You didn't do anything to become depressed. Your failure to do something didn't cause your depression. Depression is an illness. You are no more at fault for having depression than if you had asthma, diabetes, heart disease or any other illness." In other words, don't blame yourself. With the right kind of treatment nearly everyone can experience relief from depression.

Dr. Bloomfield is also one of the foremost experts on the use of herbs to treat anxiety and depression and has written two books on the subject (see Suggested Reading).

For blue moods that aren't due to the illness of depression, I recommend the following:

1. Exercise. Of course you don't feel like it! But it is nature's best road to relaxation and a more hopeful feeling. Women who exercise regularly report feeling more empowered and in control of their menopause. "When I'm on a roll with exercise, and doing it daily, if something gets in the way, and I can't do my workout, I feel sad and listless," a patient recently told me. After a business trip to Spain, which was so packed with flights and meetings she couldn't do any exercise at all, she was feeling totally out of sorts. Her experience is typical. When people who exercise daily have to stop suddenly for some reason, they often report malaise and the blues. Is it exercise withdrawal? Or is depression the natural state of human beings who go without a daily amount of exercise? From personal experience and what I've learned from my patients, I'd bet on the second.

2. If you're feeling blue because of hot flashes or other symptoms you're having a difficult time controlling, keep in mind that these uncomfortable changes are time limited. You will get through this. In fact, in most cases, these symptoms will disappear eventually, even if a woman does nothing about them. Your body will eventually achieve better balance and, with it, a less shaky sense of well-being.

3. If your trouble is mood swings, try time-released vitamin B6, also known as pyridoxine. I recommend 200 mg every day. It competes with a substance known as tryptophan for receptors in the brain and can help restore a feeling of equilibrium or, at least, take a bit off the edge.

4. Rethink your diet. Research keeps showing that there is a connection between what we eat and how we feel. The food you eat can have mental health effects. Depressed people, for example, tend to consume more sugar. These sugars supposedly spike serotonin production. And, as most of us know, a high blood-sugar level is a fast mood fix. The ups and downs of too much sugar can lead to moodiness. Try substituting more complex carbohydrates—corn, potatoes, oatmeal. They also have a calming effect, but without such an abrupt letdown because they are digested more slowly than sugar. And make sure you are getting three meals a day. You won't want to binge on quick, sugary pick-me-ups that leave you feeling tired and cranky later.

YOUR SKIN: THE NEW ABCS OF SKIN CARE—ALPHA-HYDROXY, BETA CAROTENE AND VITAMIN C

Estrogen has always been praised for its positive benefits to a woman's skin. Research shows that estrogen is partly responsible for the distribution of subcutaneous fat, which is the layer of skin that provides firmness and elasticity. It also encourages the production of collagen, which helps keep skin firm, and oils, which keep the skin from drying out. Estrogen loss, therefore, can show up in your face. However, even though estrogen replacement therapy helps you maintain these benefits, it does not turn back the clock. It does nothing about sun damage or the normal effects of aging on the face, many of which are genetic.

When you opt for Raloxifene over estrogen replacement, you may wonder if you're going to miss out on these benefits. Scientists are studying the effects of SERMs on skin, and the results are still to come. I recently asked Will Deere, head of Eli Lilly's research team on Raloxifene, when women might know if Evista would have the same effects on the skin as conjugated estrogen. He admitted that this was one of the most frequently asked questions, but the answers are probably several years away.

You are like many of my patients if you are concerned about your skin as you age and want to know what medical science has to offer you. What's working against you is sun damage and genetics.

According to dermatologists, the most well-researched news about preventing wrinkles is probably what your grandmother told you years ago when you were coating yourself in baby oil and lying in your yard with a reflector to get a deeper tan—avoid the sun. Use a sunscreen every day, at least 15, even if your day only includes going to the office. Put it on five minutes before you apply anything else to your face. Research suggests that whatever you apply to your face first is what counts. Apply a makeup base with 5 percent sunscreen and then put on the sunscreen at 15 percent, and your skin reacts to who's on first—the 5 percent.

However, there are many new advances in dermatology—the medical field devoted to skin care—that will help put time on your side. According to Dr. Darrell Rigel, Clinical Professor of Dermatology at New York University and president-elect of the American Academy of Dermatology, "The problem is that once you get to the point where you have a lot of sun damage, you really can't turn back the clock. You can stop the clock. But you can't turn back the clock in terms of what you can do for your skin."

What may help are vitamin A derivatives, vitamin C, alpha-hydroxy acids (AHAs), and mild acid peels, according to Dr. Rigel. "These simple things which are easy to do can make a significant difference in terms of how your skin appears."

Let's take a closer look at these treatments.

• **Renova—Vitamin A throws Mother Nature a curve.** Dark spots, roughness, fine lines and wrinkles—you wake up one day and notice that you definitely have them. Renova is the big news in the last few years for women past forty. It's basically .05 percent tretinoin, a retinol compound related to vitamin A. Tretinoin is the same drug that powers Retin-A, an acne medication that was rediscovered a decade ago, when it was found to also smooth the skin in older patients and help rid them of fine facial lines.

Dr. Rigel says, "The only difference between Retin-A and Renova is the base they are in. Renova is a lot less drying. The trouble with Retin-A for older women is that it is drying to the skin." Retin-A has an oil-and-water base aimed to reduce moisture in young, acne-prone skin. Renova is basically the same thing, but in an emollient base that provides added moisture.

Approved by the FDA in 1995, Renova is available only through prescription. You apply a small amount of it nightly. It takes six to ten months to work, although patients often report improvement within thirty days. Getting the fine lines to disappear takes patience—and six to eight weeks of the drug. One must continue it to keep the benefits.

There can be side effects, such as redness or irritation and peeling. Sometimes women find that using it a few times a week instead of daily helps the skin become accustomed to it. The cost is about $40 for a tube, which should last three months.

• **Retinol creams and other department store remedies—can you get the same effect from the cosmeceuticals?** The makeup industry was quick to follow the good news about vitamin A with vitamin products of its own. Department store versions can cost upwards of $60. You can get a very similar thing at the drugstore for $10, if you read your labels carefully. All these remedies contain concentrations of retinol (pure vitamin A in an alcohol form).

Are these products virtually the same as Renova or Retin-A? According to Dr. Rigel, no. "It's like saying a motorcycle and a bicycle are the same thing. They are derivatives of the same idea, but they're totally different. Retin-A and Renova are not just vitamin A. It's a different chemical. I describe it as a cousin of vitamin A."

Dr. Rigel warns that there are a lot of things out there that have been given names that sound like Renova. "They probably contain vitamin A, and the manufacturers have done different things with it, but they aren't the specific derivative of vitamin A you find in Renova or Retin-A. They are probably good moisturizers, but they aren't going to give you the same benefits of the drug itself."

In the best case, no remedy does anything for muscles that have responded to the downward pull of gravity, or drooping eyelids and jawlines. But you can probably look forward to less blotchiness and smoother, softer skin, and results after three months from Renova.

• **Alpha-hydroxy acid.** AHAs, as they are called, are found in so many skin creams today—gels, liquids, even moisturizers and makeup bases—that one can lose sight of what the hype was all about when they first came into vogue a decade ago. AHAs are usually derived from fruit, soured milk (lactic acid) or sugarcane (glycolic acid). What AHAs do is slough off dead skin cells. This makes the skin appear younger. Some researchers believe that if you continue to use them steadily, after a year they will stimulate your skin to produce structural collagen in the right places. The problem is that experts argue over what strength you need to do the trick. Most drugstore creams contain about 5 percent.

Dr. Rigel says, "A lot of the products that are out there have a pinch of alpha-hydroxy, if they even tell what the percentage of concentration is. There are different kinds of AHAs, too. If you get it from a physician, or at least from a company that you trust, you can know what you're getting as opposed to what you think you might be getting. I generally recommend women start with 5 percent glycolic and then move to 10 percent."

What's interesting is that with all the hype about AHAs, the FDA began to investigate whether they should be classified as drugs, rather than cosmetics. There's no reason not to try them, and chances are you already have a cream or moisturizer that contains AHAs. Stinging and tingling are the only known side effects.

• **Vitamin C creams.** "This was the big news in the last year," Dr. Rigel explains. "There are probably at least twenty-five versions of it out there. Vitamin C clearly has some antioxidant properties that may help with sun damage."

Advertisers of these products claim they will reduce wrinkles, firm skin and increase vibrancy. In truth, vitamin C, at a high concentration, is a natural antioxidant. Antioxidants are substances that are believed to neutralize the free radicals produced by cigarette smoke, pollution and the sun. It is said to boost the production of collagen and keep skin supple.

There are three different forms of vitamin C for the skin—ascorbic acid magnesium, ascorbic phosphate and ascorbic palmitate. Will any of them get rid of wrinkles or crow's-feet? The astounding before-and-after pictures you see in magazines may make you want to run out and buy the product, even at its cost of upwards of sixty dollars for a small bottle. At most, you can probably look forward to a freshening effect. Don't sell that short.

After a couple of months of using any vitamin C product, you should throw out what remains in the bottle. Vitamin C products become unstable quickly. When it turns dark brown, toss it. If you use the product daily and notice nothing after sixty days, you can be pretty confident that the next bottle isn't going to improve matters.

• **All-in-one facial creams.** Some of the creams available from cosmetic companies try to throw in the whole deal—vitamin C, alpha-hydroxy, high-tech moisturizers. There're little hard scientific data on these creams but enormous claims about how they can totally revitalize your skin: They remove crow's-feet. They defy gravity and make wrinkles disappear. They make you look twenty years younger. They are a face-lift in a jar. They slice and they dice! For $5.95!

You are probably going to get a little bit of everything at very low strength and a lot of emollient cream. If it irritates your skin, don't bother. Because the pH levels and acidity levels can vary greatly, you may have to try several products before you find one that feels good on your skin. If they make your skin look better in your eyes, then there is no medical reason not to use them.

• **Peeling off the years—what's new in chemical peels.** A chemical peel is an accelerated method of exfoliating the skin, which improves the quality and appearance of the skin by removing or thinning the topmost layer. There are different levels of peels. The deep peel—the phenol peel—is used very rarely. This was a very aggressive approach that left one with severely burned, crusting skin, causing very pronounced changes but at a high level of discomfort and weeks of recovery time.

Dr. Rigel recommends starting with a light acid peel. He prefers glycolic acid. "The procedure takes just a few minutes. Usually people come to see me at lunch and go back to work."

These peels regularly are performed by dermatologists but are also performed by beauty-salon technicians. There are more than nine types of peeling agents, including glycolic and lactic acids and other AHAs at different concentrations. The AHA peel you get from a dermatologist is usually in the 50 to 70 percent range of concentration. A salon usually offers a 30 to 50 percent AHA peel. The higher the concentration, the more aggressive the action. Some doctors recommend a series of peels, over a six-week period. Side effects are minimal, although swelling, flaking and redness can occur. Women who swear by them report getting rid of enlarged pores and achieving smoother coloring. Women who are disappointed complain of red skin, not unlike a medium sunburn, and dryness.

Should you go to a salon instead of a doctor for your peel? "I can't say for sure what is going on in salons," says Dr. Rigel, "but I think the difference is that what you'll get in a physcian's office is tried and true in terms of medical application. You know what you are getting. It will be stronger and more effective, because we have the ability to access those medications."

You will generally feel a stinging during a mild peel, and you will usually be told to splash cold water on your face until the stinging stops, usually five minutes. Then you will be given a moisturizer.

"A peel alone may not be enough. A regimen that includes that as well as the other topical agents, AHAs and vitamin-A derivatives and vitamin C will be beneficial. And still a woman has to protect herself from the sun. Wear that sunscreen always."

When is enough enough, in terms of a realistic skin regimen? Should you be putting as many products on your face as you can, and hope for the best. Dr. Rigel explains: "I don't tell my patients to try everything at once. Try what makes the most sense to use. Definitely start with sunscreen. Add one product at a time, such as starting with AHAs and making sure you don't have a reaction. If you try everything at once, and get a reaction, you won't know what agent you're getting a reaction to. But, yes, you can use these products in combination and see what works best for you."

• **Broad-spectrum sunscreens.** Besides the news about vitamin C, the biggest news in dermotology these days is the broad-spectrum sunscreens that have ultraviolet A protection. Dr. Rigel explains: "It's called Parsol 1789. It's in many suncreens you can buy at most drugstores and is very effective. Realize that there are three kinds of ultraviolet light. UVC has the most energy, but it's blocked out by the ozone layer. UVB are the sun's rays that burn your skin and are most often related to skin cancer. Most suncreens cover that burn well. UVA rays, however, are the less-energy, longer-wavelength rays that are involved with aging the skin. These new sunscreens are much more effective at blocking these rays."

The best skin care remedy is still diet, exercise and sunscreen. There's no question that exercise has benefits that show not only in your body but in your face. Sweating flushes out impurities, and the extra blood flow is enormously beneficial. Women who exercise regularly report better skin as well as stronger bodies. A healthy diet will also show up in your skin.

QUESTIONS WOMEN ASK

Q. If I exercise regularly with weights and take plenty of calcium, will it be enough to stop me from losing bone density?

Unfortunately, if you do not take estrogen or Raloxifene, you will still lose bone mass once you reach menopause. However, these things do help. And exercise has so many benefits, it's always a plus.

Q. I hate rigid diet plans. What's the easiest way to avoid fat and cholesterol?

Simply make your diet heavier on fruits and vegetables and lighter on meat.

natural remedies and SERMS: should you try the healing herbs?

In a health food store I visited recently, there were more than fifty remedies in the "Woman's Midlife Health" section, all claiming to do some good for women's menopausal symptoms. Are there really powders, tablets and tinctures you can buy over-the-counter in health food stores that will naturally replace the estrogen your body no longer provides? Is there a supplement that can cure annoying symptoms better than HRT and with complete safety? Is it true that remedies you can buy over-the-counter are risk-free because they come from plants? Can you take them with Raloxifene, and double the bonuses?

In short, not really. But there *are* grains of truth in every one of these statements. This chapter will help you separate what might help you from what will ultimately frustrate you and waste your money. And, if you cannot, should not, and will not take estrogen, you need to educate yourself about these botanicals, as much as you would educate yourself about a prescription drug.

IS NATURAL BETTER?

Many of my patients have growing concerns about the side effects and long-term safety of pharmaceutical drugs. They want to know, "What about a 'natural' approach to health after menopause?" Botanical remedies (over-the-counter remedies that are derived from herbs and plants) are what they usually mean by "natural." The remedies most talked about include dong quai, black cohosh, yam root and soy. These remedies have wider acceptance in Europe and many other countries, but the manufacture of "midlife supplements" is a big industry with a growing following in the United States. But before I discuss specific herbs, let me make an important point about the difference between natural and risk-free.

Natural isn't risk-free. Just because a supplement comes from plants and is available at a health food store doesn't make it safe. Granted, many of the over-the-counter botanicals are basically diluted medications that happen to come from plants, but this doesn't guarantee their safety. Herbs and extracts can be potent. All of modern medicine gets its start from plants. Digitalis, for example, is a powerful medicine that comes from a plant. But in the wrong dose, it can kill you.

In terms of HRT, there is no reason to believe any of the botanicals are preferable to medication that is FDA regulated, tested on thousands of women, and successful with millions of patients. For the most part, all we have is anecdotal evidence—women taking the drug said it helped them. Before you decide that this is enough for you, realize that we do not, for the most part, have studies comparing women taking the drug to other women taking placebos with the first group saying it helped them more. We actually have more rigorous studies comparing whether bottled water tastes better than tap water. At least the participants were blindfolded and didn't know what they were drinking.

A patient who was considering taking dong quai instead of estrogen because she was tired of suffering night sweats made worse by the summer heat told me, "I don't like the idea of taking drugs. I don't like the thought that I could increase my risk of breast cancer. I just thought this could be safer." My thought? If it's relieving your hot flashes, you can bet your liver is seeing it as estrogen even if it's called something else. And, if you think you are going to avoid the risk of breast cancer or any other side effect by using natural remedies, the reality is, if they're stopping your hot flashes, they're affecting your body, and therefore they are affecting your breasts.

They're also going to pass through your liver on the way through your body, so purity is important. These remedies are not subject to the same intense scrutiny the FDA mandates for prescription drugs. Although they are touted as having medicinal properties, they aren't labeled as such. Manufacturers are not required to test products for safety and purity.

One might wonder why the FDA doesn't step in since these botanicals are such big news and so many women are ingesting them. Prior to 1994, the FDA regulated dietary supplements much as it did foods. It evaluated the safety of all new ingredients before allowing a manufacturer to market a product, and it had the power to ensure that the health claims made by these manufacturers were truthful.

Then in 1994 the FDA lost the battle for regulation over the supplement industry. The battle was waged mainly by consumers and politicians. Analysts believe that the reason the FDA lost wasn't because botanicals are superior and "above" scrutiny but because consumers and politicians wanted the vitamin industry to go unregulated rather than lose some vitamins. It can take millions of dollars to test a supplement to the point that it achieves the standards set by the FDA, and there are many manufacturers of vitamins who are unwilling or unable financially to conduct the rigorous tests the FDA demands.

The Dietary Supplement Health and Education Act of 1994 was created following this battle. When you read the label on a supplement, you won't see claims that the supplement can prevent, treat or cure anything. Chances are what you know about a particular supplement you read in a magazine, heard from a friend or were told by the person behind the counter. The only thing supplement manufacturers can print on the label without having the FDA crack down on them is that the remedy somehow affects the function or structure of the body. In other words, the label can't say it cures hot flashes—the manufacturer has to dance around and say something such as "It promotes harmony," regardless of what it's really supposed to be doing in a woman's body. This can be confusing to a woman looking at a shelfful of "midlife supplements."

The manufacturer must also print the following disclaimer: "This product has not been evaluated by the Food and Drug Administration. This product is not intended to diagnose, treat, cure or prevent any disease." Detailed ingredient and nutritional information has to be listed on labels, but there is no way to know that what's on the label is in the bottle since the FDA doesn't have a mandate to inspect manufacturing facilities.

That said, there is definitely growing interest in botanical remedies for menopause. Keep in mind that a lot of this interest sprang up before SERMs were released. Women had fears of breast cancer and no answers from the pharmaceutical industry. Botanicals might lose the promise they once had once women realize that their doubts have been heard, responded to and developed into safer and better synthetic drugs via SERMs.

In any case, as botanicals become more popular across the

world, I want my patients to be as knowledgeable about them as I want them to be about taking Raloxifene, estrogen or any other medication. Most of these botanicals fall under the category known as phytoestrogens.

WHAT ARE PHYTOESTROGENS?

These are "plant estrogens," which appear to have plant hormones or hormone precursors in them. Although plant estrogens are very weak estrogens—the strongest is only 1/200th as strong as what your body made before menopause, according to the experts— they may perform functions that are similar. Herbalists claim that in premenopausal women phytoestrogens compete with a woman's own estrogen, reducing the total effects of estrogen. They bind to the estrogen receptors in a woman's body, competing for space with her own estrogens. The surplus of estrogen sends a chemical message to the body to stop manufacturing more estrogen. When women's production of estrogen falls at menopause, phytoestrogens supplement the hormone.

It is interesting that since the news of selective estrogens was released a couple of years ago, many supplement manufacturers suddenly are saying that their phytoestrogens are "Nature's SERMs." The components of the supplements haven't changed, just the claims. Are they merely jumping on the SERM band-wagon? This is yet to be determined.

Let's take a closer look at the most common phytoestrogens.

DONG QUAI (*ANGELICA SINESIS*)

What it is: Dong quai, or Chinese angelical root, can be taken as a pill or as a liquid that can be added to water. About thirty drops daily is the usual dose.

What it is supposed to do: It has been purported to relieve hot flashes, vaginal dryness and depression. Depending on whom you talk to, it can cure "all female complaints." An herbalist told me that it "increases the effectiveness of the estrogen that now is released primarily from a woman's fat tissue after menopause."

The bottom line: You might get a laxative effect. You might get the same amount of central-nervous stimulation you'd get from a cup of espresso. What you probably won't get is any relief from the symptoms that come with menopause. The estrogen released from a woman's fat, as claimed, is not the same as premenopausal ovarian estrogen that will protect your bones and your heart.

One controlled study, in which seventy-three women participated, showed that after six months of treatment, dong quai had no better luck banishing hot flashes than a sugar pill. As for replacing your estrogen naturally, some experts believe that dong quai actually lowers the circulating levels of estradiol. Definitely not what you need!

BLACK COHOSH (*CIMICIFUGA RACEMOSA*)

What it is: Black cohosh, also known as black snakeroot, is the root and underground stem of a North American forest plant. It grew wild in the Ohio River Valley and was used by Native American women there to relieve gynecological complaints. It is purported to supply estrogenic sterols—the building blocks for estrogen, progesterone and testosterone. Capsules and drops are the most common way women take black cohosh. The effective dose is 40 milligrams.

What it is supposed to do: Relieve hot flashes, night sweats, headaches, heart palpitations, decreased libido, depression, anxiety and vaginal dryness. The theory is that it binds to estrogen receptors, producing a weak estriol-like effect.

The bottom line: This is the best studied of the herbal remedies. European researchers report several positive studies, including one double-blind study of eighty women in Germany, where it was found to reduce menopausal symptoms better than the conjugated estrogens. There are complex chemicals called triterpenes and flavonoids, which are said to be present in black cohosh. Some studies suggest that these substances act on the pituitary gland, which is located at the base of the brain, to suppress the secretion of luteinizing hormone (LH). High levels of LH are thought to be the root of many menopausal symptoms such as hot flashes, night sweats, headaches and drying of the vagina. The German Commission E, Germany's leading authority, which evaluates the safety and effectiveness of herbal remedies, approves it for the treatment of menopausal symptoms.

It isn't cheap and you need to take two pills a day, a total of 40 mg a day, according to Germany's Commission E. Side effects that women have reported include nausea, dizziness and vomiting.

If you think it's worth a try, keep this in mind:

• There are no studies of the herb's effect when it's taken for years at a time. Germany's Commission E recommends that women use it for no longer than six months.

• I don't pretend to be an expert on herbs for menopause, nor do I recommend them to my patients, but the experts I did consult spoke most often about Remifemin as a brand of black cohosh they would recommend. I pass that information along for women who are determined to try black cohosh because while there are many brands of black cohosh available, Remifemin was used most often in the European studies where results were positive.

• Keep in mind that if black cohosh is estrogen, doctors who regularly prescribe conjugated estrogen also prescribe progesterone for twelve days each month along with estrogen to protect the uterus from hyperplasia. Women taking plant estrogens alone may run a risk of hyperplasia. If you are going to take black cohosh, don't hide the fact from your doctor and go for regular exams. Go for regular mammograms.

• I have never heard anyone even suggest that black cohosh can help prevent osteoporosis or cardiovascular disease. In your quest for relief of symptoms, don't forget the big picture.

• Don't confuse blue cohosh with black cohosh. It isn't more of the same. Blue cohosh contains caulosaponin, which can raise blood pressure and constrict the blood vessels leading to the heart. My advice is to avoid it.

CHASTEBERRY (*VITEX AGNUS CASTUS*)

What it is: Chasteberry is available as pills, tea and drops. Germany's Commission E also approves it for treating symptoms of menopause.

What it's supposed to do: Relieve hot flashes, headaches, heart palpitations and vaginal dryness.

The bottom line: Chasteberry is said to regulate hormones involved in the menstrual cycle. It is purported to inhibit the release of follicle-stimulating hormone. Supposedly, in some women Chasteberry acts like estrogen, in others like progesterone.

It may actually be a better remedy for PMS than it will be for menopause. The symptoms a woman faces when she is in the stage known as perimenopause—her body is still making estrogen but has varied supplies of progesterone because she is no longer ovu-lating regularly—may be somewhat relieved by something like Chasteberry if it does what it is claimed to do. But a woman whose body is no longer making estrogen doesn't need hormone regula-tion. She isn't making those hormones. This is part of the problem I have with health food stores lumping all these remedies together in some "female complaint" section. What a woman two years shy of the complete cessation of her periods comes in complaining of (bleeding that ebbs and flows with no regard to what day of the month it is, two-week cycles of PMS, subtle and annoying symp-toms like forgetting her brother-in-law's name) is different from what a woman may complain of when she reaches menopause (hot flashes, night sweats, a dry vagina). At their best, these remedies are not one-size-fits-all.

GINSENG (PANAX GINSENG)

What it is: Ginseng is a root that has been used in traditional Chinese herbal medicine for more than five thousand years. There are two types of ginseng: American and Chinese (or Korean). There are ginseng teas, candies and dried roots. It became so prevalent, so easily found at the checkout counter, that it wasn't long until consumer watchdog groups in the U.S. began to report that some of the over-the-counter Ginseng supplements contain little ginseng at all.

What it is supposed to do: Combat fatigue and depression, have an estrogenlike effect on the body, ease vaginal dryness and hot flashes.

The bottom line: It's probably a stimulant. In two studies in-volving more than five hundred people who received ginseng in combination with vitamins and minerals, the participants reported a boost in psychological well-being and energy. Take it as a pick-me-up and you may find that you do have more energy during the day, but you may also have lots of excess energy and anxiety at night when you're trying to go to sleep. The Asian kind is purported to be especially stimulating. If you are dealing with insomnia, irritability or anxiety, this may worsen your condition. In some women it raises blood pressure.

Though we have pretty sketchy research data, ginseng may well be a potent phytoestrogen. Women who take it have reported uterine bleeding long after they have gone through menopause. My biggest problem with ginseng is that you have no idea what dose you are taking.

WILD YAM ROOT

What it is: Also called colic root, this is a perennial plant that was once used by Native Americans to soften the pain of childbirth.

What it does: Some proponents say it can substitute for progesterone. Others say it has an estrogenic effect. Some herbalists claim that to get the best effects, you have to shave off the outer bark of the root and put the inner part in your blender to make a salve. Now here's something my patients have time to do at the end of the day when their teenagers are finally in their rooms doing God knows what, and they're trying to fix a running toilet—make salves in the blender!

One thing is for sure: You have to be highly motivated to use some of these remedies. It appears, however, that many women *are* that motivated.

The bottom line: No big surprises here. All the synthetic hormones except Premarin—including other estrogens, progesterone, progestin and testosterone—are made from wild yam root. Wild yam was once the sole source of chemicals used as raw materials in the manufacture of the birth control pill.

Women who are taking estrogen are prescribed progesterone because it protects the uterus from cancer. Sometimes the progesterone causes side effects. They may want to try yam extract in hopes of getting the benefits without the side effects. However, even though yam extract contains diosgenin, which is used in making synthetic hormones, there is no evidence that the human body can convert diosgenin to hormones as the chemical lab can. If your doctor recommends that you take progesterone and you want to go the natural route, there are many other natural progesterones on the market that will be more effective than yam root.

SARSAPARILLA

What it is: A plant that contains natural steroids.

What it is supposed to do: Relieve PMS and menopausal symptoms; be a natural source of testosterone. (Some women take testosterone after menopause to increase their sex drive.)

The bottom line: The natural steroids in sarsaparilla, which are sarsapogenin and smilagenin, cannot be converted to androgens or estrogens in the human body as they can be in the lab. The only evidence for sarsaparilla is anecdotal, and nothing in science supports its claims.

SOY

What it is: A way to change your diet during menopause, and avoid the symptoms. Asian women have a lower rate of breast cancer and report much less incidence of hot flashes than American women. When this fact was discovered, the first theory was that the difference had to do with the fact that the diets of American women are known to be high in fat. But a low-fat diet may not explain it all. Asian women regularly eat more soy products. Soy contains estrogenlike components called isoflavones.

What it is supposed to do: It may be the closest thing nature has to a phyto-serm because scientists studying the potential of soy to lower the risks of cancer, heart disease and osteoporosis believe that soy acts selectively. There have been studies that claim that women who regularly eat soy foods (twenty to forty grams of soy proteins a day) have few hot flashes and have more cells in their vaginal lining, meaning less vaginal dryness. There was also a study conducted at Wake Forest University School of Medicine, which showed isoflavones in soy proteins can lower cholesterol levels (both overall levels and the level of low-density lipoproteins or "bad cholesterol") by as much as 10 percent.

The bottom line: Can you diet your way past the symptoms of menopause? I've read much of the research about soy. It's very intriguing. The fact that women in Asia who consume a diet vastly different from that of U.S. women have less breast cancer is important. When the same women come to the U.S. and consume a Western diet, they end up with the same rates of breast cancer. We have to learn why. Is it because of a low-fat diet? Is it because these women have increased amounts of soy in their diets? It's a very intriguing idea that one can offset menopausal symptoms and health problems through diet. But it doesn't detract from the notion that if there are phyto-serms and medicinal serms, with medicinal SERMs you get quality control and you know how much you're getting. The bottom line is that there is more research needed, and it is in fact taking place. We may all have the answers within the next five years.

Many women don't want to wait. If you want to try a diet high in soy, consider that it's estimated that you need to eat twenty-five to forty-five milligrams of isoflavones a day to duplicate what Asian women routinely consume.

I'm no stranger to dieting. I know how hard it can be to maintain any special diet over months and even years. The diets I've seen that are supposed to help women through menopause and beyond are pretty stringent. Ask yourself: Can I stick to it? Can I make it a lifetime choice? In spite of my motivation to go this route, how successful have I been in the past at sticking to a diet? It's difficult in this society, where you have lunch at a salad bar and go to dinner parties, eat at airports and consume half of your food outside your home.

If your track record with dieting is sketchy and your lifestyle means you catch your meals where you can outside your home, making a commitment to a soy-based diet isn't going to be easy. Adding a little soy powder to your minestrone soup isn't the same as embracing an Asian diet. Unless you can do it all the way, you probably aren't going to get the benefits.

But, if you feel you want to give it a try, I say go for it. It isn't going to harm you. Soybeans are high in fat, but they are low in calories and do not add many fat grams to the diet. Soy milk and tempeh are strangers to most Western women's diet. As one of my patients put it, "I'd love to try this, but tempeh, even fresh, looks like leftover vanilla pudding that's beginning to do some strange metamorphosis in the fridge after a week. As far as soy milk goes, it looks like something you'd get if you milked a goat."

One needs to be very, very motivated. If you are, there is a growing list of recipe books that basically teach Western women how to hide these foods in things such as spaghetti sauce. What do you need to consume to get the same benefit Asian women get? About 120 to 150 milligrams a day.

¹/₂ cup soy milk	40 mg
¹/₂ cup tofu	40 mg
¹/₂ cup tempeh	40 mg
¹/₂ cup miso	40 mg
¹/₂ cup cooked soybeans	40 mg

RED CLOVER (*TRIFOLIUM PRATENSE*)

What it is: This plant, also called cow clover, meadow clover, purple clover and trefoil, contains 1 to 2.5 percent isoflavones (plant estrogen substances). The only dietary source richer in isoflavones is soy.

What it's supposed to do: Reduce menopausal symptoms; add estrogen to the body "naturally."

The bottom line: Something that looks promising is Promensil, an extract of red clover that is being actively marketed for menopause symptoms. The manufacturer of Promensil has tried to counter the charges against supplements (i.e., no clinical tests and no uniform dosage) by subjecting Promensil to rigorous testing and safety standards and promoting it as a standardized source of isoflavones. The forty-milligram tablet contains four isoflavones in a standardized amount and ratio. To get the same amount from a diet, the manufacturers note that a woman would have to consume eight cups of chickpeas and a cup of soy milk—a whopping 2,000 calories.

Two placebo-controlled clinical trials involving ninety-eight perimenopausal women revealed no adverse side effects after three months of treatment. None of the women experienced uterine bleeding over the course of the study, and vaginal ultrasound performed in forty-three women showed no evidence of endometrial thickening.

The recommended usage is one tablet per day. This amount of estrogenic isoflavones is intended to equal the amount one would get in a typical vegetarian diet or Japanese diet.

The jury is still out. It may be worth looking into. Read the literature on it.

SHOULD YOU TAKE THE SO-CALLED HEALING HERBS WITH RALOXIFENE?

I've had patients who are having some transitory hot flashes in the beginning of their Raloxifene treatment, or encountering vaginal dryness, who want to know if they should supplement their Raloxifene with some herbal remedy. Until I hear research that makes me believe differently, if these supplements are estrogen, then they are being seen by your breasts as estrogen and your liver as estrogen, regardless of what they are called and there is no definitive research that shows any of them to be selective.

Much of the excitement about phytoestrogens came before the release of Raloxifene, when women had little choice but to take synthetic forms of estrogen and be concerned about its effect on their breasts or to go without it entirely. Now that Raloxifene looks so promising, taking phytoestrogens may hold their appeal only for women who have a deep mistrust of synthetic drugs. In my opinion it doesn't make much sense for a woman to bypass the advantages of protecting herself from osteoporosis, or reducing high cholesterol and breast cancer, just to take something that is called "natural" but is in fact medication. They may bring relief now but leave you unprotected against the most life-threatening problems post-menopausal women face. As far as wanting something derived from a plant is concerned, Premarin is the only synthetic estrogen that isn't from a plant. But, most important, is that you don't definitely avoid any negative effects of estrogen with the phytoestrogens.

The alternative products may work best for mild symptoms. In terms of hot flashes, avoiding obvious triggers, dressing in layers and exercising may help you just as much if your symptoms are mild.

HOW TO HAVE A SAFE VISIT TO
THE BOTANICAL PHARMACY

I'm no stranger to health food stores. There are vitamins I buy regularly I wouldn't do without. But to guard yourself against needless expense and possible health hazards, keep the following in mind:

• Clerks who give you advice may have good intentions, but they are not pharmacists, do not undergo any special training to hold their jobs and should not substitute for your doctor. Do your own research. And don't feel you shouldn't tell your doctor what you're taking or planning to try. A good doctor isn't there to judge you but to help you achieve the best health possible.

• Avoid the combination products. There are a lot of "midlife" remedies out there that try to stuff everything that might help into one bottle. Remember that menopause has its stages—perimenopause, early menopause and late menopause. They are not all the same, because the body is making different levels of hormones at each stage. Remedies that contain a little ginseng, a little black cohosh, some of this and some of that scare me. If there is a list of ingredients, there's probably too little of anything to make a difference. But throwing combinations of medications into your body is a setup for problems. And why take something that is basically a remedy for menstrual cramps when you're no longer menstruating?

• Don't believe that this is the quick path to recovery. Women who report benefits often have been taking a particular supplement for four weeks or more. In any case, if you are taking a supplement to alleviate symptoms and see nothing happening after a couple of months, why bother?

QUESTIONS WOMEN ASK

Why are doctors so hung up on double-blind studies? Maybe medical science is being blind. Thousands of women say that something they can get in a health food store helps them with hot flashes. If it's been used in ancient medicine since before most of us were born, and it works, what more do we need to know?

Don't be taken in by the words *ancient* and *traditional,* as if anything that was manufactured in the last decade is no good. Modern medicine has the best record when it comes to saving lives. No research can dispute that. With all the hype about "natural remedies" these days, the most frequent complaint I hear from patients trying to soothe their symptoms with botanical remedies is that they don't give much relief from anything that they can tell. The truth is that tablets marked "Ancient Remedy" are often bestsellers in the U.S. when research shows that, across the world, people are turning away from traditional treatments and embracing modern medicine.

What more do you need to know in terms of taking the so-called phytoestrogens? I think you need to know more than whether or not they will relieve a hot flash. If a substance I am swallowing is going to be ingested and absorbed systemically, then I would want to know what dosage it is and what safety and purity I can be assured of since the substance will pass through my liver. Women need to ponder whether it will cause the endometrial lining to proliferate, increasing the risk of cancer. When doctors prescribe synthetic estrogen for women, progesterone is also prescribed. How are you going to supplement that, or deal with this possible effect, if these phytoestrogens do in fact act like estrogen? In which tissues is it acting like estrogen; in which tissues is it acting like an estrogen blocker? We don't know. You may hear a lot of raves, but the truth is, we have no better research on these products than we do on thigh cream, which as one of my patients put it is "All show and no go."

Are there any drugs in nature that can relieve hot flashes, preserve bone and be antiestrogenic in the breast and uterus? If they exist, they would put us one step closer to synthesizing such substances in the laboratory.

My doctor pretty much rolls her eyes when I tell her about wanting to try phytoestrogens. I'm about ready for my annual exam, and I've been taking some of these supplements for a couple of months. Should I mention that?

I would advise any woman who wants to try over-the-counter remedies not to keep her doctor in the dark. If these remedies help you, good. Just make sure that they are not harming any other part of your system at the same time. Get regular checkups. Are you suddenly having vaginal bleeding? This could mean that what you're taking is, in fact, acting like estrogen in that it is causing endometrial stimulation. Again, nature can be potent.

When I tell my friends I'm taking estrogen, they look at me like I'm unevolved or something. I wasn't one of the lucky ones. Teas and tinctures and all that stuff cost a fortune, and weren't doing much from what I could tell. Why is there such a big debate between women who take herbs and women who take synthetic drugs when we're all pretty much in the same boat, trying to feel better?

You can come to feel from all you read in magazines about what natural remedies might promise that you're somehow a better person if you can achieve your goal of getting through the problematic points of menopause through diet instead of medicine. That's stretching it, given the stakes here. It's hard enough in this society with the stresses and expectations of career, of family, of self just to find enough time to exercise, keep yourself fit and eat well. Most of us take vitamins, or supplements, but turn to synthetic drugs to protect our health when the risks are high not because we're lazy but because we are realists. Do what's most realistic for you. Do what will be most beneficial to your health.

If double-blind placebo-controlled studies are the answer to knowing whether these products work or not, why isn't someone doing them?

Pharmaceutical companies know that when they believe they have a marketable drug, rigorous scientific trials have to follow to bring it to market. It's a long, costly road. These studies can take ten years or more to complete. To get a drug through the research phase, through three or more individual experimental trials that ready it for a final submission to the Food and Drug Administration, can cost up to $500 million.

Drug companies are public companies that have to be profitable to their stockholders. It's true that if there is no profitability, drug manufacturers might not pursue something my patients might be interested in. But at the same time these companies help humanity. Who else has the motivation and means to bring drugs to market? Like it or not, profit has been the motivation for a host of wonderful discoveries in the last decade.

Do I wish there were somebody altruistic enough out there who could answer the questions my patients have about botanicals and donate billions of dollars to research without any promise of a return on their dollar? Definitely. Do I see anyone out there doing it? Unfortunately, no.

SEVEN

raloxifene, tamoxifen and beyond: preventing breast cancer through SERMS

On Monday, April 6, 1998, I went to my health club as usual and got there about a quarter to seven in the morning. I began to ride the exercise bike in front of the TV that is tuned to the *Today* show each morning. For the first fifteen minutes of the show, they aired the story of a new "wonder drug." "For the first time," they claimed, "it has been shown that a drug could actually prevent breast cancer." I was in absolute shock and amazement because the drug they were describing was Tamoxifen.

If you or someone close to you has had breast cancer, chances are you've heard about Tamoxifen or Nolvadex, its trade name. Developed in 1966 and approved by the FDA in 1978, Tamoxifen is approaching 10 million women-use years of experience as adjuvant (i.e., additional) chemotherapy following surgery and/or radiation for early-stage breast cancer. It is the most widely prescribed antineoplastic drug and has saved countless lives.

Seven years ago, the media also dragged it through the mud. Tamoxifen was actually the first SERM. Early research showed it was a potent antiestrogen in breast tissue. Cancers that appear to depend on a supply of estrogen to grow were cut off from the natural supply. In addition, long-term use of Tamoxifen produces estrogenlike effects that maintain bone density and lower circulating cholesterol and LDL cholesterol. Some studies show a reduction in heart disease from the use of Tamoxifen as well. However, Tamoxifen had been around for almost ten years when news that it might have a side effect of causing uterine cancers began to surface. Dr. Maureen Killackey, then a gynecologic oncology fellow at Memorial Sloan-Kettering in New York, made the first report of three patients with adenocarcinoma of the uterus who were receiving "antiestrogens" (the term that was once applied to the drug Tamoxifen). Later, in 1988, a series of letters to the editor, mainly of the prestigious British journal *Lancet*, showed up discussing the association between Tamoxifen and uterine cancer. The first scientific prospective study was published in 1990 by Patrick Neven in Brussels, where he followed sixteen patients for three years using hysteroscopy. The incidence of uterine cancer was 6 percent; polyp formation 25 percent; and stimulation of uterine endometrium 43 percent. Only 50 percent of patients, in other words, did not experience an adverse effect in the uterus from Tamoxifen. Studies I published supported Neven's study and described a 30 percent incidence of polyp formation, a 13 percent incidence of uterine stimulation with or without precancers and a 4 percent incidence of uterine cancer in women receiving Tamoxifen.

However, seven years ago when these studies were making big news, I appeared on national public radio and local CBS radio pleading with women who had breast cancer to stay on their Tamoxifen because it will save lives and prolong lives in women with breast cancer. These women had to understand the math: Many more women were going to die of recurrences of breast cancer without Tamoxifen than were going to die from uterine cancer with it. (I will discuss this in depth later in this chapter.) I had many patients who had been treated for breast cancer, were survivors and felt very vulnerable, very worried about ever having to go through any kind of cancer scare again. But the numbers simply didn't justify walking away from something that was going to save their lives.

This, then, was the same Tamoxifen, dragged through the mud by the media only seven years before. Used for more than twenty-five years to treat breast cancer, the real news was that Tamoxifen could also be enlisted to *reduce* breast cancer. Science had finally proved that such a thing could be done. Breast cancer reduction had become a reality, and it wasn't because of a vaccine as many had thought it would be, but a category of drugs known as SERMs.

What the *Today* show as well as news programs and papers across the country reported was information from the Breast Cancer Prevention Trial (BCPT). The trial was studying whether Tamoxifen could prevent breast cancer in women who are at increased risk of developing the disease. It involved 13,388 women, all of whom were at increased risk of developing the disease, either because of their age or other factors. The study had been stopped fourteen months earlier than planned because it showed such a dramatic reduction in breast cancer risk among women taking Tamoxifen compared to those taking a placebo that they felt it was unethical to continue the study in its present format. They wrote to the women who were part of the study explaining why they were stopping it. One of the women shared her letter with *The Philadelphia Inquirer* that Sunday, and by Monday morning it was all over the airwaves.

To understand the ramifications of stopping one of these studies midstream, which actually happens quite frequently, imagine that you're a woman at risk for breast cancer, either because of family history, or just because of your increasing age, which is actually the biggest risk factor of all. You decide to become part of a study in which a drug is going to be tested to see whether or not it helps prevent breast cancer. When the study involves taking medication, you are made well aware at the start that the drug in question is not proven, or that there's no definitive knowledge about whether you might experience side effects. You also know that you may get the drug or you may get a sugar pill.

Thus it was with the trial of Tamoxifen. Beginning in June 1992, a total of 13,388 participants were recruited and randomized to receive either a placebo or Tamoxifen. The average amount of time on the drug was 3.6 years. It was a study of high risk with "high risk" defined as either being over age sixty or having one or more first-degree relatives with breast cancer.

There are advisory groups who watch these studies carefully. In the case of the Tamoxifen study, the advisory board was the NSABP (National Surgical Adjuvant Breast and Bowel Project). When the study was into its sixth year and this advisory board saw a 45 percent decrease in breast cancer among women taking Tamoxifen, they said in essence, "Wait a minute. This is so significant, it's not fair to women in the study taking nothing, since all of these women are at significant risk. We have to notify them." The rest is history, via *The Philadelphia Inquirer* and *Today*. Before a formal release of any data, the whole world was watching.

My concern—and I got the opportunity to voice it when I was invited to appear on a CNN special about breast cancer that evening—wasn't that there was good news about Tamoxifen, but the fact that no one was saying that Tamoxifen was one of a category of compounds known as SERMs. The other two are Toremifene, marketed under the trade name Fareston for metastatic breast cancer, and Raloxifene, marketed under the trade name Evista for prevention of postmenopausal osteoporosis. No one was mentioning that there were other SERMs that might have similar effects and perhaps be even safer. Although there was a 45 percent reduction of cases of breast cancer among those taking Tamoxifen, there was also a 240 percent increase in the number of cases of uterine cancer in patients on Tamoxifen versus those on a placebo—a number that rises to 433 percent if you look only at postmenopausal women. In addition, 55 percent of Tamoxifen-treated patients described vaginal discharges, of which 12 percent described them as bothersome.

About a month later, Eli Lilly released its own data on Evista and breast cancer prevention at a meeting of the American Society of Clinical Oncologists. In one study of 7,704 women with osteoporosis on Raloxifene to see if it would reduce the incidence of fractures (a treatment study), there was a 74 percent reduction in breast cancer in these women, whose median amount of time on the drug was twenty-nine months. Furthermore, this was the first report showing a trend toward a reduction in uterine cancer of 62 percent in patients taking Raloxifene compared with those given a placebo.

At that same meeting pooled data from 14,800 patient years' cumulative exposure to Raloxifene—and this included women in osteoporosis prevention as well as osteoporosis treatment studies—showed there was a 58 percent reduction in new-onset breast cancer compared to those women on placebo alone.

That was major news. After two years, their clinical data already showed great effectiveness. But there was one problem in comparing the two. The Tamoxifen study was done on women at high risk for breast cancer. The Raloxifene study was done on healthy postmenopausal women who were being studied for the drug's effect on their bones. The incidence of breast cancer was recorded as a "secondary end point," something that is studied and quantified even though it's not the purpose of the study. Critics say the Tamoxifen study had been looking at high-risk women. However, it's not as if we're comparing apples and oranges here. We're comparing two SERMs, quite similar, both of which are potent antiestrogens in the breast. The point is that one of them—Raloxifene—does not cause adverse effects in the uterus.

Many women ask me this: "Isn't it necessary to study Raloxifene for ten years before declaring it to be safe, since it took almost ten years of use of Tamoxifen before the association with endometrial cancer was appreciated?

The answer is no. It does not take ten years for Tamoxifen to cause abnormalities in the uterus—we see these within the first twelve months of use. It is because the incidence of these abnormalities is relatively low and therefore it took that long for anyone to appreciate any cause and effect or link between taking the drug and developing uterine cancer.

THE SAFER SERM

Although Raloxifene is newly released, it isn't a newly invented drug. The drug was around as far back as the early 1980s. It was being tested at the M.D. Anderson Hospital from 1982 to 1986 as a breast cancer drug. It performed very similarly to Tamoxifen, a drug that was and still is marketed to breast cancer patients. It performed no better than Tamoxifen, so the drug was put on the shelf. Who was going to spend a fortune developing a drug that offered no more benefits to women than an existing drug?

In the late 1980s and early 1990s when news surfaced that Tamoxifen causes a very small but increased risk of cancer of the uterus, interest in Raloxifene was renewed. Why? Scientists suddenly remembered one of the more interesting findings during the early studies of Raloxifene, a finding that suddenly had major ramifications: its total lack of any stimulatory effect on the uterus.

Most of us know, of course, that before a drug is tested on human beings it undergoes extensive testing on laboratory animals, usually rats. There is no such thing, however, as a postmenopausal rat. In order to do experiments on these animals, the scientist has to remove ovaries from the rat, which renders it postmenopausal. It had already been shown that Tamoxifen could stimulate the endometrial lining to proliferate in such rats. But this was not the case with Raloxifene—it was a pure estrogen blocker. It did not stimulate the uterus at all. In other experimental animal studies, Raloxifene had been shown to prevent bone loss, reduce serum cholesterol and be a potent antiproliferative on breast tissue.

Although the experimental animal data looked hopeful, what would happen in women? If Raloxifene were to be Tamoxifen-like in the uterus of postmenopausal women, then it would offer no advantage. If, however, it was a pure estrogen antagonist in the uterus while maintaining the same beneficial SERM profile in bone, lipid and breast as Tamoxifen, this drug could be a home run for women—the bonuses of estrogen without its risks. Eli Lilly wanted to be sure that they didn't have another Tamoxifen—good for one cancer, risky for developing another.

In May 1995, I received a phone call from a research physician at Eli Lilly. "Dr. Goldstein," he said, "you know as much as anyone in the world about looking at the lining of the uterus with ultrasound. Will you help us develop some studies of uterine safety for a new compound?"

Although I was well-known for my work in gynecologic ultrasound, I had never before done any work with a pharmaceutical firm. I was at the point of declining when he told me who else was going to be on the Gynecology Advisory Board, including physicians like Malcolm Whitehead from England and Patrick Neven from Brussels. These were world-famous luminaries, doctors I had often quoted in my lectures. I couldn't resist.

The compound they were studying was, of course, Raloxifene. The way scientists have always studied whether a drug has the potential to develop cancer of the uterus is to perform a uterine biopsy on women and see if there is any abnormal tissue. A uterine biopsy is an office procedure in which a catheter is passed into the uterus and a small sample of tissue is taken from the lining. I don't want to frighten women, but if a woman goes to be tested with a biopsy, biopsies get about 4 percent of the uterine surface area. If you have an abnormality that involves only a portion of the lining, or is in a polyp, a biopsy could miss it completely. I conducted a research study of 433 perimenopausal patients with abnormal uterine bleeding. It was demonstrated in that study that an office biopsy alone would have potentially missed polyps, submucus fibroids and hyperplasia (precancer) in up to eighty patients or 18 percent of the time.

Our gynecology advisory group devised a protocol for a specific study to look at Raloxifene and uterine safety. This study used transvaginal ultrasound, saline infusion sonohysterography and endometrial biopsy at frequent intervals.

By the time I was called in, there were already some ongoing studies. In one interim analysis of 136 patients in which treatment with Raloxifene, in a relatively high dose, was compared with standard continuous combined hormone replacement therapy, there was no stimulation of the uterine lining, no polyp formation, no hyperplasia in the Raloxifine group, but there was 30 percent stimulation of the lining, 3 percent polyp formation, and no hyperplasia in women undergoing continuous combined HRT. In addition, about 9 percent of the patients on continuous combined HRT discontinued the study because of bleeding, while no one in the Raloxifene group did. That study, which was not as thorough as the one I subsequently helped to design with the gynecological advisory board, had powerful enough results, however, that I felt totally comfortable that it proved that even in the first year, Raloxifene was *not* Tamoxifen-like in the uterus. I presented those data at the North American Menopause Society in September 1997. I was also with Eli Lilly at the FDA advisory hearing panel, invited so I could speak to the uterine safety issue, which was the paramount concern.

Recently the ultimate uterine safety study I helped design was completed. It showed no polyp formation, virtually no proliferation, no hyperplasia (precancer), cancer, and no tissue buildup on either transvaginal ultrasound or saline infusion hysterography.

SHOULD YOU BE ON A SERM?
IF SO, WHICH ONE?

Fareston is for metastatic breast cancer. Tamoxifen has been approved for adjuvent chemotherapy for women with breast cancer and, as this goes to press, is on the brink of being approved for prevention of breast cancer. Raloxifene is for virtually all postmenopausal women, because they are all at risk for osteoporosis.

There are different groups of women who may be pondering their treatment options in the next decade: the group that has already had a bout with breast cancer; has been treated for it; and has taken, is taking or has been advised to take Tamoxifen. Another group is those women who have strong reasons to want to prevent a breast cancer and would consider daily medication to lower their risk. A third group is women who are not at particularly high risk for breast cancer but who are disinclined to take medication to preserve bone or lower cholesterol, etc., because of concern about long-term effects of such drugs on their breasts and uterus.

• **The breast cancer survivor—which SERM is for you?** If you fall into this category, your primary question may be: Is Raloxifene better than Tamoxifen at preventing a recurrence of my breast cancer? You can begin to consider whether or not it's better for you by answering the following questions:

Have you had a hysterectomy? If you have, then the fact that Tamoxifen might increase chances of uterine cancer is a moot point for you. If you still have your uterus, then this potential side effect is something you have to consider. Don't mistake an "increased chance" for "If I take Tamoxifen I'm definitely going to get uterine cancer." The numbers of women who develop cancer precursors is relatively small, and Tamoxifen saves lives.

Have you been through your five years of Tamoxifen therapy and wonder what you should do next? You probably know that five years is the recommended course of Tamoxifen treatment. The data show that Tamoxifen does not decrease recurrence of breast cancer after five years. Nor is survival increased after five years. That is why the National Cancer Institute does not recommend using Tamoxifen after five years. It is not because it has been proven dangerous after that length of time. It is because it no longer does what it is indicated to do. However, breast cancer in the contrelateral breast was decreased in patients on Tamoxifen between five and ten years.

Many women do go longer with supervision from their doctors.

It is their form of HRT for their bones and lipids, since most will not consider estrogen. With the recommendation from the National Cancer Society that one should discontinue Tamoxifen after five years, Raloxifene makes the most sense. I can't recall a patient of mine with breast cancer who has been willing to take estrogen. Many stayed on Tamoxifen for longer than five years because prior to the release of Raloxifene, they really had no other alternatives for HRT.

• **You want to prevent breast cancer—is Tamoxifen or Raloxifene the answer?**

When the stories broke about Raloxifene and Tamoxifen, there was a lot of discussion on television and radio about what women, who had no real risk of breast cancer but fears of it, would make of this news. Would they go running into their doctors' offices asking for this preventive drug? Would it be ethical for doctors to prescribe it for them?

When this book went to press neither drug had been approved by the FDA for this purpose (although by the time you read this, is it likely that Tamoxifen will have been approved). Can you get a prescription anyway? Yes. Your doctor can prescribe it "off label." What that means is once a drug is FDA approved, a doctor can prescribe it if he or she thinks it will help a patient, regardless of what it is specifically indicated to treat. It's not that unusual. Think of how many women were prescribed birth control pills to treat acne.

There's no question that the healthy woman who is looking for a preventive agent has the trickiest choice. There's Tamoxifen on the one hand, with twenty years on the market, and now Raloxifene, with three years of data. They've both been studied for a brief time as preventive agents.

It is true that the cancer scare with Tamoxifen has been over-dramatized. But, it's also only the tip of the iceberg. Research shows that women taking Tamoxifen have a 25 percent to 30 percent incidence of polyp formation and a 13 percent to 18 percent incidence of hyperplasia (precancers). Almost 50 percent of women who take Tamoxifen can be expected to manifest these abnormalities, but the majority will be benign.

The if-you-get-it-we-can-treat-it philosophy sounds great on paper. Until you meet women who come in with one of these uterine scares, it's difficult to fathom how traumatic it can be. It often requires undergoing a D&C. It often means days of stress and tension.

I've had two patients with breast cancer who recently faced this predicament. The first patient, who had taken Tamoxifen for just over a year said, "There's no way I'm going to continue to take this drug!" She already had one malignancy (breast), and now she had a scare in her uterus—a large polyp. I removed that polyp, which was benign. But she had no intention of continuing Tamoxifen. Rather than have her take nothing, I encouraged her to opt for Raloxifene.

The second patient, who also had a Tamoxifen-induced benign polyp, was more focused on the fact that she hadn't had a recurrence of breast cancer with Tamoxifen. She decided that with careful monitoring she could continue. Neither woman is right or wrong—they are just making decisions that make sense for them.

What I am recommending to the healthy woman who wants to preserve bone, lower cholesterol **and** prevent breast cancer is Raloxifene. While it is true that six years and $50 million have been spent studying Tamoxifen, six years ago Tamoxifen was the only available SERM to study. We don't have six years' worth of data on Raloxifene with breast cancer as a primary end point in highest-risk women. What we do have is petri dish data, which I'm comfortable saying are just as good as Tamoxifen's. We have experimental animal data that are just as good as Tamoxifen's and three years' worth of data showing a reduction ranging from 58 to 74 percent versus six years' worth of data showing 45 percent reduction.

Real women with real problems need solutions. If you are a fifty-two-year-old woman and both of your sisters and your mother had breast cancer and you want to go on an agent to reduce your risk of breast cancer, I would recommend Raloxifene over Tamoxifen (if you have a uterus). Raloxifene does not stimulate the uterus. It does not cause uterine cancer. It does not cause polyps, it does not cause precancers and it does not cause bleeding. In fact, it seems to lower your risk of uterine cancer.

What I tell my patients is, "If you start this drug today, you start with three years of data. In two years, there will be five years of data. You aren't hooked into taking it forever. If longer-term data are your only real concern, you will have them shortly."

The best news about Raloxifene and the reduction of breast cancer is for those women who are not taking HRT because of fear of breast cancer but who are not really at high risk. If these data on Raloxifene's reduction in breast cancer risk will allow you to comfortably take this drug, then the benefit to your bones and your lipid profile and thus, perhaps, your heart, breast and uterus is multiple. The use of Raloxifene for women to preserve their bone mass and as a by-product getting a significant reduction in new-onset breast cancer (not to mention the reduction in cholesterol, the lack of uterine bleeding and/or potential uterine cancers) makes this an easy recommendation.

In a couple of more years, as we'll discuss in the next chapter, you may have even more SERMs to choose from and the very likely possibility of individualizing treatment options for various women through SERMs.

Are there any other potential side effects of Tamoxifen?

Yes. Most commonly, hot flashes (30 percent), sweating (17 per-cent), nausea (15 percent), and vaginal discharge (16 percent). Blood clots are also a side effect, just as they are with estrogen and Raloxifene. During the BCPT study, two women died from pulmonary embolism (blood clot in the lung) and both were in the Tamoxifen group.

Can I really eliminate my chances of ever getting breast cancer with Raloxifene or Tamoxifen?

What we are really talking about is risk reduction, not elimination. You should be aware of the fact that these chemopreventative agents will significantly reduce your risk of breast cancer but not eliminate it. You cannot forgo breast examinations or mammo-grams. You should remain a nonsmoker and stay on a low-fat diet.

In the study that showed Tamoxifen could reduce breast cancer risk, you note that the women were all high risk. What criteria were used to determine high risk?

Women over age sixty were allowed to participate, regardless of any other factors, because age is the biggest risk factor. Women thirty-five to fifty-nine had to prove they had other high-risk fac-tors, including a primary family history of breast cancer (a mother, sister or daughter diagnosed with it); a history of breast lump biopsies; early-age onset of menstruation; and late-age delivery of first child, or no natural children.

Are minority women regularly included in any of the studies of Raloxifene or Tamoxifen?

Yes. During the Tamoxifen study, for example, special efforts were made to recruit minority women, including a public service announcement featuring singer Nancy Wilson. An outreach program to businesses and churches in communities where large numbers of minority women reside was also utilized.

EIGHT

medicine in the
new millennium

At this moment, scores of scientists around the world are in their laboratories trying to create the ideal SERM. This SERM will be the one that stops the hot flashes; prevents breast cancer and osteoporosis; gives youthful benefits to the skin; provides protection against heart attacks, Alzheimer's disease, blood clots and more. An impossible dream?

We began this exploration of SERMs with the dilemma of estrogen. Women's longevity has gone through the roof in the last 150 years. There are tissues in the body where the presence of estrogen has tremendous benefit as women live longer. Estrogen's definite benefits include preserving bone health, lowering cholesterol and apparently preventing heart disease. There's also the possible maintenance of cognitive function and a reduction in Alzheimer's disease, as well as benefits to skin and connective tissues. However, there are other tissues—the breast, the uterus, the venous system with potential for blood clots—that do not want or need an estrogen function. Up until now, a woman has had to confront either putting estrogen in all the tissues of her body and gaining its benefits in spite of the risks, or forgoing estrogen and trying to maintain her health through a variety of natural approaches and lifestyle choices.

This book has been the story of SERMs (Selective Estrogen Receptor Modulators). SERMs have the potential to extend postmenopausal women's health. Tamoxifen, first developed as a drug to fight breast cancer, was found to possess estrogenic properties in bone preservation, fracture reduction, lipid lowering and heart attack prevention. It was the first SERM, even before scientists realized that there was such a category of compounds.

Raloxifene is a second-generation SERM that comes from a benzothiopene derivative. Its foremost improvement over Tamoxifen is that it has no deleterious effect on the uterus in postmenopausal women. Early reports also seem to indicate that women experience less intensity, severity, and duration of hot flashes as well as much less incidence of discomforting vaginal symptoms when taking Raloxifene, compared with Tamoxifen.

What can women look forward to in the next decade? Drug companies are not always forthcoming with information on what they have in development; these are public companies whose stock prices can shift on rumor as well as reality. But here is some of what we know:

- Levormeloxifene, from the European company Novo Nordisk, is not a Tamoxifen analogue but is structually similar to Centchroman, a drug used as an oral contraceptive in India since the late 1980s. It appears to have a favorable SERM profile, closer to Raloxifene than that of Tamoxifen.

- Droloxifene (Pfizer), a Tamoxifen analogue, is in clinical trials.

- Idoxifene (SmithKline Beecham) is being tested as an anti–breast cancer drug but is also being investigated as an osteoporosis drug.
- CP-336,156 (Pfizer) is a compound being tested for protection against osteoporosis and heart disease.
- SERM3 (Eli Lilly), is the name the company that manufactures Raloxifene has given to its next Selective Estrogen Receptor Modulator. This is said to be similar to Raloxifene but more potent with a main thrust toward preventing breast cancer.
- Wyeth-Ayerst, the maker of Premarin, is working on its own SERM in cooperation with Ligand Pharmaceuticals.
- Zeneca, the maker of Tamoxifen, has some pure anti-estrogens in the pipeline. These would be strictly for advanced breast cancer.

How close are we to the perfect SERM? Dr. V. Craig Jordan is director of the breast cancer research program at Northwestern University Medical Center in Chicago and one of the foremost experts on SERMs; he is often called the "Father of Tamoxifen" for his contributions to that drug's release. He thinks it's very possible in our lifetime. "Think of penicillin. Back in the 1940s, we're in a wartime situation and there are huge numbers of casualties. Scientists are wondering, 'What's our best bet to try to develop something to be able to stop all of these war wounds from killing the soldiers so we can get them to recover?' They go back through the literature and find this unknown agent that has some positive activity in animals. It's penicillin. The pharmaceutical industry develops it, but it doesn't work for everybody. It only works on certain bacteria. But it opens the door to the antibacterial age. It gives a whole new dimension to therapeutics. Now we can selectively kill bacteria that cause certain diseases that have been killing patients for generations.

"Today we have a whole spectrum of antibiotics, dozens and dozens to choose from. I think of Tamoxifen as the penicillin in a war that's been against breast cancer. The focus was: 'Do something about breast cancer, find a preventive.' When Raloxifene followed Tamoxifen, a broader-spectrum use of this drug class began that will now open the door for future SERMs that will perhaps prevent coronary heart disease, Alzheimer's and more. If we can find out how these things work, we can continue to produce drugs that have multiple positive effects for women. Women, for the first time, now with this new era have choices they've never had before as more of these agents get onto the market."

SERMs AND BEYOND: MEDICINE IN THE NEW MILLENNIUM

Doctors are men and women of science who, for the most part, get uncomfortable when asked to guess or make predictions about the future. But I feel comfortable enough from my own research and from studying the research of my colleagues to make a few predictions about what will occur in the field of women's health over the next decade. Here is what I think you can safely count on:

• I believe there will be third- and fourth-generation SERMs that will increase the benefits of estrogen while continuing to diminish the risks. All this will extend postmenopausal women's health. Perhaps we will see the development of SERMs for men. Men could use some cholesterol reduction, prevention of heart attacks, prevention of Alzheimer's and preservation of bone mass. The effect of such compounds on the prostate gland in particular will be something more scientists will become interested in over the next ten years.

• Scientists will grapple with the challenge of seeing if they can create a hormonal milieu in postmenopausal women that will be even more beneficial than that produced by normal, functioning ovaries in younger women. This means studying what other substances may be involved and at what levels. We may find that some of the "natural" ovarian hormone production is actually detrimental, as your own natural estrogen may be for your breasts or unopposed estrogen is for your uterus. The concept of SERMs applied to younger women may allow us to do better than nature itself.

• Herbal and so called "natural" treatments for medical ailments of menopause will come under more intense scientific scrutiny. You will no longer have to rely on anecdotal evidence. If something works, you'll have an understanding of why and how it works. Double-blind studies, mostly in Europe, are in progress now on many of the more popular herbal remedies. If these remedies stand up to the scientific method, doctors will have more alternatives to offer patients. Concerns about humanistic and holistic approaches and the ability to marry these with modern medicine will increase. I believe traditional medicine will merge with the best of natural remedies. Doctors will know when nature will do it best; naturalists will know when we must circumvent nature to do what's best for the patient.

• You will live longer. Life expectancy has increased in the last 150 years because of such things as vaccines, antibiotics and water purification systems. There will be a major emphasis on increasing the quality of life as we age.

• Menopause will not be the end of your childbearing years. Various forms of assisted reproductive technologies will allow women over fifty to have children if they desire them and are willing to utilize high-tech procedures. Baby-boom women who once debated whether or not they should prevent conception will find themselves in an even hotter debate about whether or not to continue it indefinitely.

• There will be much less invasive surgery. Better diagnostic procedures, mainly from routine use of ultrasound in the gynecologic exam, will make many invasive biopsies and exploratory surgeries obsolete. Increasingly gynecological procedures will be done endoscopically through the laparoscope and hysteroscope.

• My final prediction is this: Menopause, as a psychological concept, won't have nearly the negative connotation it's had in the past. Women will view it as the beginning of a new phase, rather than the end of anything. With so many women living thirty, forty and even fifty years postmenopause, the whole idea of "the change" really becomes just that—a change, rather than an affliction. Healthy, vital, fifty-something, sixty-something and seventy-something women will be looked to as role models by younger women. *Isn't she something? What did she do to feel so great at that age that I should be doing?*

Perhaps in our youth-centered society these women will never be as revered as they are in ancient cultures. But they will be admired for their fortitude. Their persistence and unwillingness to accept menopause as a disease will cause many a medical breakthrough as they demand answers. They will be copied and studied. Their senior years will become a time of greater purpose and growth unparalleled by any generation before them, and they will make their mark.

In closing, my central message to you is this: In balance, hormone replacement therapy is beneficial. Even if there is a slight increase in breast cancer—and I'm not even a hundred percent sure that there is, although I too recognize the possibility of some link existing after long-term use—the balance sheet in terms of health benefits, quality of life and longevity clearly favors being on hormone replacement therapy. Having said that, those of my patients (and currently the majority of my patients) who will never, ever touch hormone replacement therapy because of fears of breast cancer as well as those who tried it and stopped because they didn't feel good finally have an option. We're still a decade away from the best SERMs have to offer, but for your best health, I would rather see you on a SERM than on nothing. I believe it is your best bet for long-term postmenopausal health.

Those of you who are doing well on estrogen, even if you have a few nagging questions in your mind about it, also have an option. You needn't switch to a SERM immediately. Wait awhile. See what other data we get about estrogen and Raloxifene. See if science develops third- and forth-generation SERMs that are even better.

If statistics are correct, 80 percent of women are scared off and doing nothing in terms of estrogen replacement. If having this new option of SERMs makes that percentage come down, we will go a long way to extending postmenopausal women's health.

As you grapple with the realities of menopause, remember that knowledge is power. My hope is that you will take that power and use it to create not only longevity but also a finer quality of life.

suggested reading

Could It Be . . . Perimenopause? Steven R. Goldstein, M.D., and Laurie Ashner. New York: Little, Brown, 1998.

Endovaginal Ultrasound. Steven R. Goldstein, M.D. New York: John Wiley & Sons, 1991.

Estrogen: The Facts Can Change Your Life. Lila Nachtigall and Joan Rattner Heilman. New York: HarperPerennial, 1995.

How to Heal Depression. Harold H. Bloomfield and Peter McWilliams. Los Angeles: Prelude Press, 1995.

The Lotte Berk Method. Lydia Bach. New York: Random House, 1973.

Menopause and Midlife Health. Morris Notelovitz, M.D., and Diana Tonnessen. New York: St. Martin's Press, 1993.

Managing Your Menopause. Wulf H. Utian and Ruth S. Jacobitz. Paramus, NJ: Prentice Hall, 1992.

The Relaxation and Stress Reduction Workbook. Martha Davis, Ph.D., Elizabeth Robbins Eshelman, M.S.W., and Matthew McKay, Ph.D. Oakland, CA: New Harbinger Publications, 1988.

The Silent Passage: Menopause. Gail Sheehy, Julie Rubenstein (editor). New York: Pocket Books, 1993.

When Is Enough, Enough? What You Can Do If You Never Feel Satisfied. Laurie Ashner and Mitch Meyerson. Center City, MN: Hazelden, 1997.

Women's Primary Health Care: Office Practice and Procedures. Vicki L. Seltzer, M.D., and Warren H. Pearse. New York: McGraw-Hill, 1995.

index

Acetylcholine, 12
Acne, 104
Alesse, 70, 73
Alpha-hydroxy acid, 134
Alzheimer's disease, 12
    lowering risk of getting, 115
    and Raloxifene, 77–78, 104–5
Antidepressants, 128
Antioxidants, 134–35
ApoE4, 77
Assisted reproductive technologies,
    180
Aygestin, 22

Bach, Lydia, 122
Bellergal, 110
Birth control pills, 34–35
Black cohosh, 144–46
Blood clots, 51, 95
Bloomfield, Harold H., 129
Blue cohosh, 146
Bone
    and estrogen, 14–16
    loss, 66–67, 96
    and Raloxifene, 41–44
Breast cancer, 2, 8, 33–34
    and HRT, 25–28, 97
    and Raloxifene, 47–49, 68–69, 75–77

SERMs for prevention of,
    169–71
SERMs for survivors of, 168–69
Breast Cancer Prevention Trial, 161
Breast tenderness, 105

Caffeine, 33, 123
Calcium, 14, 43, 116–17
Centers for Disease Control, 26
Chasteberry, 146–47
Chemical peels, 136–37
Cholesterol
    and estrogen, 11, 97
    and Raloxifene, 44–45
    remedies for lowering, 113–15
Chopra, Deepak, 125
Climara, 20
Clonidine, 110
Coffee, 33
College of Physicians and Surgeons
    (Columbia U.), 12
Commission E (Germany), 145
Complex carbohydrates, 130
Contraception, 27
Corpus luteum, 45
CP-336, 156, 177
Creams, 21
Cummings, Steven, 69

Deep vein thrombosis, 51
Deere, Will, 131
Depo-Provera, 112
Depression, remedies for, 126–30
DEXA test, 67–68
Diagnostic and Statistical Manual of Mental Disorders, 127
Dietary Supplement Health and Education Act (1994), 142
Dieting, 119
Dong quai, 143–44
Double-blind studies, 155–56
Droloxifene, 176

Eli Lilly, 163, 165
Emotions, 16–17
Endometrial proliferation, 94
Estrace, 20
Estraderm, 20
Estradiol, 71
Estring, 21, 63–64
Estrogen, 1, 5–9, 45–46
  and Alzheimer's disease, 12
  and bones, 14–16
  and cholesterol, 11, 97
  complaints about, 21–24
  concerns about, 19
  disenfranchisement from, 62–63
  and emotions, 16–17
  and hair, 18
  and heart disease, 10–11, 97
  and hot flashes, 12–14, 110
  and libido, 17–18
  and longevity, 14
  receptors, 9
  and skin, 18, 130–31
  skin patches, 20–21
  and sleep, 18, 122
  tablet form, 20
  and teeth, 19
  vaginal inserts, 21
  and youthfulness, 89
Estrogen Lite, 53
Evista. *See* Raloxifene
Exercise, 32, 87, 116, 129

Facial creams, all-in-one, 135
Fans, 111
Fareston, 167
FDA
  drug approval, 42, 55
  regulation of natural remedies, 140–42
Fibrinogen, 44
Flexibility, 121
Fosamax, 43, 92, 98–99, 102
Free epinephrine, 13
FSH (follicle-stimulating hormone), 13, 34, 71–72

Ginseng, 147–48

Hair, 18
  loss, 105
Half-life, 92
Halfpapp, Elisabeth, 120–21
HDL cholesterol, 11, 44, 114
Healing herbs. *See* Natural remedies
Heart disease, 10–11
  and estrogen, 10–11, 97
  risk factors for, 74–75
Heel bone scan, 68
High blood pressure, 88–89, 101–2
Hot flashes
  and estrogen, 12–14
  and Raloxifene, 49–51, 53–54, 63–65, 100–101
  remedies for, 109–12
How to Heal Depression (Bloomfield & McWilliams), 129
HRT, 5–9, 54–55, 59–60, 70
  and breast cancer, 25–28
  complaints about, 21–24, 69–70
  continuous-combined, 46–47, 96, 167
  cost of, 86
  dosage and forms of, 19–21
  questions about, 30–35
  sequential, 22, 95–96, 106
  side effects of, 97
Hyperplasia, 48
Hypothalamus, 109

Idoxifene, 177
Insomnia, 18
    remedies for, 122–26

Jordan, V. Craig, 56, 69, 177
*Journal of the American Medical
    Association*, 27

Killackey, Maureen, 160

Lancet, 26, 160
LDL cholesterol, 11, 44, 114
Leg cramps, 51–52
Levormeloxifene, 176
LH (luteinizing hormone), 73, 145
Libido, 17–18
Life expectancy, 8–9, 29, 179
Loestrin, 70, 73
Longevity, 14
Lotte Berk Method, 120–22
The Lotte Berk Method (Bach), 122
Lunch, 123–24

McWilliams, Peter, 129
Megestrol, 110
Men, 106–7
Menopause, 1
    average age of, 103
    future connotation of, 180
    remedies for, 109–38
    stages of, 71–74, 154
    surgical, 13–14
    symptoms of, 49–51, 54, 96
Muscle building, 120–22

National Cancer Institute, 76, 168
National Institutes of Health, 28
National Osteoporosis Foundation,
    15
Natural remedies, 139
    black cohosh, 144–46
    chasteberry, 146–47
    dong quai, 143–44
    and FDA regulation, 140–41, 179
    ginseng, 147–48

questions about, 155–58
and Raloxifene, 153
red clover, 152–53
safety concerns, 154–55
sarsaparilla, 149
soy, 149–52
wild yam root, 148–49
New England Journal of Medicine, 14, 26,
    110
Night sweats, remedies for, 109–12
North American Menopause Society,
    126
NSABP (National Surgical Adjuvant
    Breast and Bowel Project), 162
Nurses' Health Study, 10–11, 26, 28,
    97

Ogen, 20
Oily skin, 104
Oral contraceptives, 73–74
Osteopenia, 15
Osteoporosis
    and estrogen, 15–16
    and Raloxifene, 23–24, 33, 42, 75,
        98–99
    remedies for, 115–17
    risk factors for, 66–67
    testing for, 67–68
Ovarian tumors, 58–59
Ovaries, 13

Parsol 1789, 137
Peak bone mass, 14
Perimenopause, 71–74
Period (menses), 22–23, 95–96
Philadelphia Inquirer, 161–62
Phytoestrogens, 143–57
Pre-existing medical conditions, 23
Premarin, 20, 105, 153
Prempro, 22, 46–47, 88, 100–101
Prevention, 66
Progesterone, 21–22, 31, 46
Progestin, 112
Promensil, 152
Prometrium, 22

Provera, 21, 94–95
Pyridoxine, 130

Raloxifene (Evista), 1–2, 29, 37, 176
  and blood clots, 51
  and bones, 41–44
  and breasts, 47–49
  and cholesterol, 44–45
  comments about, 92–94
  cost of, 86
  development of, 163–67
  how to take, 91–92
  ideal candidate for, 62–70
  and leg cramps, 51–52
  and men, 106–7
  and menopausal symptoms, 49–51
  misconceptions about, 53–55
  and natural remedies, 153
  non-ideal candidate for, 70–79
  questionnaire, 79–87
  questions about, 55–60, 87–89,
    94–107, 172–73
  safety of, 57–58
  trials, 40–52, 75
  and uterus, 45–47
Red clover, 152–53
Remifemin, 145
Renova, 132–33
Restful Sleep (Chopra), 125
Retin-A, 132
Retinol creams, 133
Rigel, Darrell, 131–37
Ring, 21

St. John's Wort, 128
Sarsaparilla, 149
SERMs, 1, 29, 37, 61. See also
    Raloxifene
  action of, 56–57
  benefits of, 38–39
  for breast cancer prevention,
    169–71
  for breast cancer survivors, 168–69
  defined, 39–40

in future, 175–81
revolutionary aspects of, 1–2
Serotonin reuptake inhibitors, 128
Sexual interest, 17–18
Side effects, 24
Skin, 18
  patches, 20–21
  remedies for, 130–38
Sleep. See Insomnia
Sodium, 120
Sound Soothers, 124
Soy, 149–52
Stroke, 32
Sugar, 130
Sunscreen, 131
  broad-spectrum, 137–38
Supracervical hysterectomy, 103
Surgical menopause, 13–14

Tablets, 20
Tamoxifen (Nolvadex), 75–76, 99–100,
    159–73, 176
Teeth, 19
Today show, 159, 161–62
Transvaginal ultrasound, 99–100
Triglycerides, 44

Upset stomach, 102
Uterus
  cancer of, 2, 45
  and Raloxifene, 45–47
UVA rays, 137
UVB rays, 137
UVC rays, 137

Vaginal dryness
  and estrogen, 17–18
  and Raloxifene, 49–50, 53–54,
    106
  remedies for, 112–13
Vaginal inserts, 21
Vitamin A, 132–33
Vitamin B$_6$, 130
Vitamin B complex, 110